The Hospice Companion

Best Practices for Interdisciplinary Assessment and Care of Common Problems During the Last Phase of Life

The Hospice Companion

Best Practices for Interdisciplinary Assessment and Care of Common
Problems During the Last Phase of Life

Perry G. Fine, MD

Professor of Anesthesiology
Pain Research Center
University of Utah Medical School

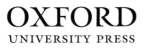

OXFORD
UNIVERSITY PRESS

2008

OXFORD
UNIVERSITY PRESS

Oxford University Press, Inc., publishes works that further
Oxford University's objective of excellence
in research, scholarship, and education.

Oxford   New York
Auckland   Cape Town   Dar es Salaam   Hong Kong   Karachi
Kuala Lumpur   Madrid   Melbourne   Mexico City   Nairobi
New Delhi   Shanghai   Taipei   Toronto

With offices in
Argentina   Austria   Brazil   Chile   Czech Republic   France   Greece
Guatemala   Hungary   Italy   Japan   Poland   Portugal   Singapore
South Korea   Switzerland   Thailand   Turkey   Ukraine   Vietnam

Copyright © 2008 by Oxford University Press, Inc.

Published by Oxford University Press, Inc.
198 Madison Avenue, New York, New York 10016

www.oup.com

Oxford is a registered trademark of Oxford University Press

Library of Congress Cataloging-in-Publication Data
Fine, P. G. (Perry G.)
Hospice companion : best practices for interdisciplinary assessment and care of common problems
during the last phase of life / Perry G. Fine.
     p. ; cm.
Includes bibliographical references and index.
ISBN 978-0-19-536997-7
1. Hospice care—Standards—Handbooks, manuals, etc.   2. Palliative treatment—Standards
—Handbooks, manuals, etc.   3. Terminal care—Standards—Handbooks, manuals, etc.   I. Title.
II. Title: Best practices for interdisciplinary assessment and care of common problems during the last
phase of life.
[DNLM: 1. Hospice Care—methods—Handbooks.   2. Palliative Care—methods—Handbooks.
3. Patient Care Team—Handbooks.   4. Terminally Ill—psychology—Handbooks.   WB 39 F4952h
2008]
R726.8.F553 2008
362.17'56—dc22   2008006739

9 8 7 6
Printed in USA
on acid-free paper

Acknowledgments

The Hospice Companion is the synthesis of many dedicated individuals' efforts. It has been prepared to reflect the fundamentals of hospice as an integrated and comprehensive system of expert-level palliative care at the end of life as we progress into the 21st century. In order to meet the goal of excellence in end-of-life care is a *rule* in our society, not an *exception*, this manual is dedicated to all those who continually strive for improvement in end-of-life care. I am especially grateful for the time and effort contributed by Dr. Todd Cote, for suggesting improvements. And, as ever, it bears endless repetition that the real debt of gratitude for the inspiration and motivation behind works such as this belongs to the patients and those at their bedsides who know the true value of *companionship.*

About the Author

Perry G. Fine, MD is a professor of anesthesiology in the Pain Research Center, School of Medicine at the University of Utah in Salt Lake City. He was the medical director of the first Medicare-certified hospice in Utah two decades ago, and subsequently he served as the founding National Medical Director of VistaCare, where he authored the VistaCare incarnations of *The Hospice Companion*. Subsequently, he served as the Vice President for Medical Affairs and Senior Fellow for Medical Leadership at the National Hospice and Palliative Care Organization. Currently, Dr. Fine chairs the National Initiative on Pain Control and serves on the Boards of Directors of the American Academy of Pain Medicine, the Society for Arts in Healthcare, and the American Pain Foundation.

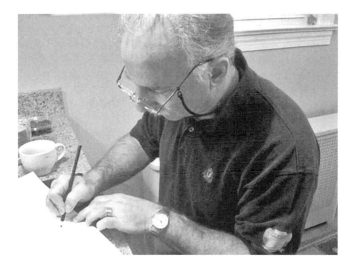

Foreword

With the publication of *The Hospice Companion*, it is again timely and important to reflect upon and to celebrate our many successes in medicine. In the United States, we have created a society where the majority of those born into it can expect to live a long and relatively healthy life. In equal measure, though, we need to be mindful of where there is room for ready improvement. This self-same world, abounding in highly technical interventions to restore function and prolong life, also seems to conspire to make the inevitable process of our dying inhumane.

A high priority goal in health care as we mark this milestone in our societal calendar is to consolidate our knowledge and processes of care into a system of care that provides comfort and dignity to all during the last phase of life. Of equal importance is the necessity of using our resources wisely so that all may benefit from the most appropriate types of care in the most reasonable and desirable setting based upon the circumstances we face as individuals. Clearly, high-quality palliative care and hospice need to be folded into the usual continuum of care—something that has yet to occur. These approaches to health care need to be seen for what they really are: optimal care for individuals with incurable illness.

The first step toward this "normalization" and eventual integration process is credibility among health care professionals and value by the public. For these to occur, foundations need to be laid for a standard of care, following the model established for so many other domains and "niches" of health care. *The Hospice Companion* is intended to serve as a guide, through which many of the processes of end-of-life care can be learned, emulated, and measured, thereby establishing standards.

The content of *The Hospice Companion* is based in the science of methodologically sound study wherever possible. Since much in the realm of symptom management has not undergone the rigors of randomized controlled clinical trials, recommendations made in the text for comprehensive biomedical, psychosocial, and spiritual inteventions/support are based upon exigent literature and the summary input of many of the most experienced hospice professionals in North America.

In its aggreggate, this manual should provide members of the interdisciplinary team insight into each discipline's particular role and foster clinical integration and enhanced communication. An effort has been made to be comprehensive, but it is recognized that the content of this manual is not exhaustive—future editions will benefit from suggestions made by those who use this one, but an effort has been made to keep it compact enough to retain its portability for bedside use. It is equally recognized that very real time limitations and other practical constraints preclude exhaustive investigation and application of the extensive "Findings" and "Processes of Care" provided in *The Hospice Companion* for all patients and situations where they might apply. They do serve to remind hospice care providers of what can be done and then to prioritize their time accordingly.

Finally, it is with an ever-deepening sense of humility, joined hand in hand with the muse of divine irony, that compels me to conclude: *It will be through disciplined clinical conformity and uniformity of practice that individual epiphany may have the chance to be realized as we meet our earthly ends.*

Perry G. Fine, MD, Center Ossipee, New Hampshire and Salt Lake City, Utah

Preface

Clinical Excellence, Innovation, and Comprehensive Palliative Care for All Patients at the End of Life

The Hospice Companion is introduced with a highly charged and unwavering goal: to promote, establish, maintain, and continuously improve comprehensive systems of care that ensure the highest quality of services to meet the needs of patients and their families during the last phase of life. On behalf of their patients, all hospice providers must inculcate processes of care that lead to maximal comfort and functional capacities and a sense of being valued throughout the final stages of any chronic and progressive illness. The values embodied in *The Hospice Companion* reflect a commitment to these premises:

- The dying patient's achievable goals are the highest priority of care.
- Family preferences are respected and supported whenever possible.
- All terminally ill patients and their families deserve access to hospice care.
- Ongoing investment to advance the art and science of palliative care is a moral imperative.
- The spirit of hospice as the most humanistic form of care at the end of life must be continually nurtured through interdisciplinary work.

We must continually recall and recommit to the core values that fostered the birth and ongoing genesis of hospice. This work is grounded in a comprehensive view of health care, in recognition that human beings are not merely sapient biological entities. During illness, physical, emotional, and spiritual needs, especially at the end of life, all require and deserve attention and nurturing. Whereas emotional and spiritual needs have not really changed much over the many years that humans have consciously grappled with mortality, medical science has evolved dramatically in the last few decades since the inception of hospice care in the United States and its coverage for the majority of those with end-stage diseases through the Medicare Hospice Benefit.

Therefore, more than ever, it is incumbent upon those who provide care to those with life-limiting illnesses to be keenly aware of both the extent and the limits of the technological advances that can add either great burden or great benefit to seriously ill patients and their families. Benefits include our much enhanced ability to relieve physical suffering, especially pain, and, in an ever-increasing number of cases, an increased capability to extend life without adding to those individuals' sense of suffering. Burdens, on the other hand, include assailing patients and their loved ones with false hopes for recovery, the imposition of costly and low-yield therapies, and technologically aided prolongation of the dying process without attention to the suffering experienced by the patient and the family when there is no hope of meaningful recovery.

Balancing the assets and liablilities of our application of modern medical science to the dying is, and will continue to be, an ongoing challenge. This balance
must be continually struck on a case-by-case basis, working ethically and in
good faith to communicate clearly and with due regard for the inevitable biases
of our own particular points of view. It is a matter of great importance to our
national public health that everyone who has chronic progressive disease or is
otherwise facing a terminal illness is aware of the options that exist in order to
make truly informed choices about what can be done to complete their lives in
comfort, no less achieve their particular attainable life goals. This is a realizable
dream. This type of care can—and should—be available to everyone who
wants it, without forcing people to give up any form of care that has a reasonable likelihood of adding quality or quantity to remaining life.

Toward this end, all hospice programs need to be committed to what has
been called "open access," providing the full measure of palliative care to all
those with a limited prognosis who elect hospice care. In view of the multiple
and various definitions of the term "open access," herein I will use the term
"comprehensive palliative care" to imply the full range of coordinated and interdisciplinary services that address patient and family needs during the last
phase of life. It should be noted that in this definition there is no mention of restrictions based upon technology or cost. These pragmatic issues must be managed and reconciled through benefit-burden analysis on a case-by-case basis,
clinical proficiency building for complex case management within hospice programs, and mastering sound business practices. In so doing, the real focus of
care will remain patient/family-centered and access to needed services will not
be restricted for any reason, other than a patient's well-considered determination that she or he simply does not want what hospice has to offer. Through
this philosophy of hospice care, and keeping abreast of all developments that
may enhance the quality of life of patients with far advanced disease, it is my
goal to set the stage for an era of even greater humanism as our society, led by
the "Baby Boom" generation, moves forward into the 21st century. It is my enduring hope that a philosophy of comprehensive palliative care, coupled with
the newly designated medical subspecialty of hospice and palliative care, will
bridge the extensive gap that currently exists between what most people currently experience during the last months of life and what is indeed possible.

The Hospice Companion has been created to operationalize the mission and
values of modern-day hospice through the individual and combined efforts of
our most valuable asset, you, the hospice professional! The title word "*Companion*" was expressly chosen for the profound meaning it suggests: that companionship, in the many forms it can take, is the key ingredient to care. No
quality or quantity of resource material can ever substitute for the company
you keep with those who are dying. That said, presence alone, although always
necessary, is seldom sufficient to meet the needs of the dying and their families.
It is what we do, as well as when and how we do it, at the patient's bedside that
distinguishes hospice as a comprehensive program of care during the last phase
of life. This book represents the practical embodiment of the basic, fundamen-

tal elements of care, through a focus on common problems confronting patients, their families, and their caregivers.

The Hospice Companion is intended as a guide through which some mastery over the seemingly complex, challenging, and oftentimes chaotic world of advanced disease may be derived. Use of this "tool" to direct processes of care during the intense interpersonal experiences of hospice work should allow the greatest opportunity for personal and professional growth and a deeply gratifying sense of accomplishment as you proceed in the all-important work of caring for the dying.

What is *not* included in this manual is equally important to mention. Absent are in-depth guidelines, content, policies, or procedures related to palliative (oncological) chemotherapy, artificial nutrition and hydration, ventilatory support, advanced management of heart failure (i.e., inotropic or mechanical support), palliative sedation, or pediatric palliative care. These (and no doubt other topics of great importance for select patients) are all very important topics worthy of separate and detailed treatments, but they are beyond the scope of this foundational manual whose intent is to address most peoples' circumstances most of the time. It is my thesis that if the vast majority of hospice providers could demonstrate mastery over the processes of care within this manual, as evidenced by measured positive outcomes, then both the credibility and overall quality of hospice care in America would be greatly improved.

Contents

Section One: General Processes 1

Palliative Care at the End of Life: Blending Structure and Function 1

From Information to Care 1

Balancing Benefits and Burdens of All Interventions 6

The Interdisciplinary Team 7

Addressing Needs Over Time 10

Documentation 15

Section Two: Personal, Social, and Environmental Processes 19

Abuse in the Home 19

Advance Care Planning and Directives for Healthcare Interventions 21

Changes In Body Image and Loss of Independence 23

Changes in Family Dynamics 25

Completing Worldly Business 28

Controlled Substances: Misuse and Abuse 30

Cultural Differences: Respect, Understanding, and Adapting Care 32

Denial 34

Grief Reactions 35

Living Environment, Finances, and Support Systems 40

Basic Home Safety 41

Suicide: Risk, Prevention, and Coping When It Happens 44

Section Three: Clinical Processes and Symptom Management 49

Air Hunger (Dyspnea) 50

Agitation and Anxiety 56

Anorexia and Cachexia 61

Belching and Burping (Eructation) 63

Bleeding, Oozing, and Malodorous Lesions 66

Confusion/Delirium 70

Constipation 74

Coughing 77

Depression 79

Diarrhea and Anorectal Problems	82
Dysphagia and Oropharyngeal Problems	85
Edema: Peripheral Edema, Ascites, and Lymphedema	88
Fatigue, Weakness (Aesthenia), and Excessive Sedation	91
Fever and Diaphoresis	93
Hiccups	95
Imminent Death	97
Insomnia and Nocturnal Restlessness	101
Nausea and Vomiting	105
Pain	108
Pruritus	128
Seizures	130
Skeletal Muscle and Bladder Spasms	133
Skin Breakdown: Prevention and Treatment	135
Urinary Problems	140
Xerostomia (Dry Mouth)	143
Section Four: Appendices	145
Appendix 1. Palliative Radiation Therapy in End-of-Life Care: Evidence-Based Utilization	145
Appendix 2. Principles of Pharmacotherapy	153
Appendix 3. Ketamine Protocols	156
Appendix 4. Clinical/Functional Assessment	161
Appendix 5. Palliative Performance Scale (PPS)	162
Index	163

Section 1

General Processes

Palliative Care at the End of Life: Blending Structure and Function

From Information to Care

The overarching purpose of this manual, reflecting the essential goals of hospice, is to help maximize the quality of living and dying of patients during the last phase of life. With due regard for the complexities of peoples' lives, especially during severe illness, it is premised that identification and understanding of discrete situations (interwined and enmeshed as they may be) will promote the elaboration of a care plan that will have the greatest likelihood of meeting these worthy ends.

A sequential system of reasoning and problem-solving is required, and this has been devised using a standardized format throughout each subsection related to symptom management (Section Three). To accommodate the interdisciplinary nature of hospice care and promote use of this manual by all members of the interdisciplinary team (IDT), headings have purposefully been chosen that reflect a common language for all disciplines. In full appreciation of the complex and irreducable nature of human dying, an organized structure is nonetheless useful to define the mechanics and fundamentals of hospice care and the overall goal of making high-quality interdisciplinary care during the last phase of life the rule, rather than the exception.

The overall schema is summarized below. This is followed by an elaboration of terms and concepts used throughout *The Hospice Companion.*

It is recognized that variables such as advanced stage of disease at the time of hospice admission, often with very short survival times, may severely curtail the range of services that might otherwise be useful to patients and families if they had the benefit of an earlier referral with a resultant longer length of stay. In many cases, the processes of care in this book might appear to be idealized because so many patients are referred to hospice just before they die. Therefore, the full range of evaluation, assessment, and interventions proposed may need to be changed in order to hone in on the highest priorities of the patient and family to meet their most pressing needs before death. At the time of admission, attention to the likely longevity of the patient (i.e., prognosis) needs to be well considered so that the issues and goals elaborated in this guide might be realistically and specifically tailored to the needs and attainable goals of each and every patient.

Basic Steps: Taking Care of People Who Are Dying, and Doing It Well

The flow chart (Figure 1.1) depicted in this section defines the essential steps that need to be followed, or at least considered, in the process of caring for patients at the end of life. It also serves as a teaching tool and reminder of the fundamental goals of patient-centered care within a larger system of health care. Last, it should help unravel the complex nature of the care system, clearly defining steps along the way that lead to successful patient outcomes and professional gratification.

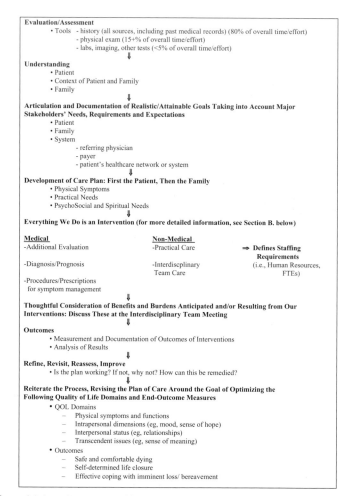

Figure 1.1 Logical progression of hospice case management.

The role of hospice is to deliver the most effective end-of-life care in the most efficient manner possible to all dying patients.

Principles of Effective Care

- The patient defines what help is needed and wanted. However, counseling about what is possible and realizeable is critically important because many patients and families will be unaware of the scope of hospice services.
- As a hospice professional, know what you can contribute to accomplish these goals.
- Know who to call upon when you reach the limits of your capabilities.
- Think and act positively. "Can't" or "Won't" are not helpful.
- Actively listen: this is a powerful tool for understanding others, validating peoples' needs to be understood, and planning and providing care.
- Define *benefits* and *burdens* for each proposed therapeutic intervention (note: advising, counseling, and taking a "watch-and-wait" approach are all forms of an "intervention" and in this vein should be viewed in equal regard as medical treatments), remembering that there are distinct points of view: patient, family, other caregivers, professional staff, and other "stakeholders" [e.g., payer(s)]. Ask and answer: What is each party hoping for? What are the underlying motivations?
- *Benefits* and *burdens* are context driven, requiring a full understanding of each patient's clinical and social circumstances. Determine in advance how benefits and burdens will be assessed, how often, and by whom. If *burdens* can be anticipated (e.g., constipation from an opioid analgesic), how can they be minimized in order to amplify benefits?
- Set priorities by determining which issues are most pressing.

Principles of Efficient Care

- Time is the most precious commodity we have. It must be allocated wisely and well.
- More goods (durable medical equipment, supplies, drugs), in and of themselves, do not equal better service or care. Determine what and how much of these items are necessary to accomplish the patient's goals, and continually reevaluate if they are doing what is intended.
- Clinical managers/leaders should cross-train and schedule human resources wisely. Determine how members of the IDT can meet patient/family goals, both to utilize their unique skills and to distribute work in an equitable and optimal fashion.

Terminology and Organizational Elements Used in Sections 2 and 3 of This Manual

Sections 2 and 3 of this manual will be structured in a similar manner as a means of reinforcing interdisciplinary, comprehensive care. Depending upon relevance, most, but not all, sections will include every dimension of assessment and process of care.

Situation

Every patient/family comes to hospice with unique attributes, clinical circumstances, and social contexts. The process of elucidating those situations that affect the well-being of each patient/family is critical to the provision of good care.

Causes

Most troublesome situations encountered by hospice patients/families can be traced to a single dominant cause or multiple contibutory causes. These causes usually stem from one or more of the following domains:

- Practical (i.e., environmental, financial)
- Biomedical (i.e., disease-induced or treatment-related etiology)
- Psychosocial (i.e., related to interpersonal or intrapersonal issues)
- Spiritual (although not always easily defined in words, spiritual concerns often revolve around issues of one's sense of purpose, existence, or meaningfulness, in life and after death)

For the purposes of this guide, causes will be identified for those medically induced symptoms for which a differential diagnosis is important in the consideration of medically specific treatments.

These listings of causes are not meant to be all-inclusive but rather to provide the leading or first-line and secondary causes for most symptoms.

Findings

Findings are those elements (usually *symptoms* [patient report] and *signs* [information obtained by observation or examination] that define or accompany any given situation and may help to identify the cause(s) of that situation. Findings are also categorized as Practical, Biomedical/Physical, Psychosocial, or Spiritual. These findings serve to identify, direct, and focus processes of care.

Assessment

The initial and ongoing determinations of Psychosocial, Biomedical/Physical, and Spiritual findings involve information gathering from one or more of the following three basic domains:

- History

  Information obtainable from all sources (medical records, interviews with patient, family members, other caregivers) is far and away the most time-consuming and important part of evaluation.

- Physical Examination

  This component of assessment involves observation of patient, family and environment, and hands-on examination of the patient.

Albeit essential for accurate diagnosis, physical examination also links the patient and caregiver through human touch, which has therapeutic value in and of itself. Needless to say, only skilled and appropriately licensed clinicians should be involved in physical examination of the patient.

- Diagnostic Studies (blood work, imaging, other)

  These types of corroborative studies are often unnecessary in order to provide high-quality palliative care at the end of life; however, there are circumstances where clinical impressions derived from history and physical examination are insufficient to formulate a well-conceived care plan. Under these circumstances, the potential benefits need to be weighed against the actual or likely burdens.

Processes of Care

The interventions listed within this section define those actions that might be taken by the IDT in order to meet patient/family needs and goals, identified through sufficient assessment.

Goals and Outcomes

Establishing goals at the outset aligns the patient/family/hospice team and promotes the monitoring of the most relevant outcomes. By explicitly stating goals, the IDT can continually assess the value of the work being done, and determine if the Plan of Care is appropriate. Anticipation of eventualities and putting contingency plans into place are critically important to delivering high-quality end-of-life care. Ideally, outcomes will match the goals that are identified. In other words, the closer outcomes are to goals, the more successful hospice care has been.

Documentation and Medical Record

Guidance is provided in the crucial areas of Initial Assessment, Interdisciplinary Team Notes, and IDT Care Plan in order to promote concise and pertinent record keeping. Thoughtful consideration of what needs to be documented serves the dual purposes of meeting regulatory compliance standards and helping the IDT to continually rethink and revisit issues that arise or are likely to arise in the context of any given patient/family system.

The Practical, Biomedical, Psychological, and Spiritual Dimensions of the Human Experience

The many inseparable dimensions of the human experience cannot be so readily categorized or unintegrated, especially under the circumstances of facing the end of one's life. As important as it may be to acknowledge this, it is equally important to identify and meet the various needs and attainable goals of dying patients and their families, with the hope that each individual can find meaning and value in her/his life as that life comes to a close. From this pragmatic starting point, four axes, or dimensions, have been used in *The Hospice Companion* to sort out and understand the nature of FINDINGS, ASSESSMENT, and PROCESSES OF CARE. **It is critically important for the IDT to understand that these dimensions do not delineate lines of inquiry or intervention by specific disciplines but rather those facets of the patient's or family's experience for which discrete aspects of the Care Plan can be formulated and carried out and outcomes can be measured.**

Practical

These are the everyday, fundamentally important things that surround our lives, most of which we take for granted while we are healthy and able to care for ourselves.

Biomedical

This aspect of end-of-life care addresses the impact of disease on the human body and those tools that modify, reverse, slow, or palliate the progression/consequences of these inevitable biological processes. A depth of clinical knowledge, judgment, and experience is needed to understand and appropriately apply modern medical interventions in ways that will best serve the various needs and goals of patients at this stage in their life.

Psychosocial

Psychological, emotional, and social issues constitute the intrapersonal and interpersonal nature of human existence. These issues are highly complex even under the least stressful circumstances and become the focus of most need once basic physical symptoms are brought under control. Attention to these issues in ways that speak to the needs of dying patients and their families is implicit to quality hospice care.

Spiritual

Ultimately, one's sense of connection, meaning, purpose, or value within the greater scheme of things is most likely to rise to the surface when confronting mortality. Attention to this uniquely human concern, at the pace and within the framework of the patient/family ethos, presents a truly marvelous opportunity for everyone involved and distinguishes hospice care from other alternatives within the health care system.

Balancing Benefits and Burdens of All Interventions

Because assessment and treatment approaches offer a mixture of possible benefits and burdens to the patient, which vary depending upon each patient's circumstances, considerable thought is needed to attend the best means to optimize benefits, while minimizing burdens. The following stepwise outline should help facilitate this process (see Figure 1.2).

First

Prior to all medical procedures, all psychosocial or diagnostic tests, prescriptions, and spiritual care interventions:

- Review pathophysiology and prognosis of ongoing disease.
- Review family structure, support, beliefs, culture, and community ties.
- Review options for palliation of symptoms tailored to the medical/social context of the patient.
- Consider comorbidities and impact of treatment choices.

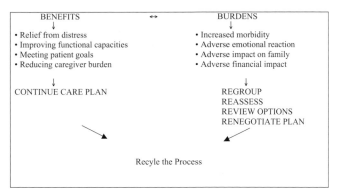

BENEFITS	↔	BURDENS
↓		↓
• Relief from distress		• Increased morbidity
• Improving functional capacities		• Adverse emotional reaction
• Meeting patient goals		• Adverse impact on family
• Reducing caregiver burden		• Adverse financial impact
↓		↓
CONTINUE CARE PLAN		REGROUP
		REASSESS
		REVIEW OPTIONS
		RENEGOTIATE PLAN

Recyle the Process

Figure 1.2 Assessing Benefits and Burdens

Second

- Discuss plans and options with patient, family, and referring physician in the context of patient's goals.
- Anticipate and discuss benefits and burdens.
- Initiate preventative strategies to minimize likely burdens (e.g., drug-related side effects).

Third

- Monitor and assess impact of intervention
- Weigh benefits versus burdens

The Interdisciplinary Team (IDT)

The Functional Hospice IDT

While there are many elements that contribute to an exceptional hospice, the interdisciplinary team is at its core. In fact, the interdisciplinary rather than multidisciplinary nature of hospice is what distinguishes it from conventional health care delivery structures. The more typical multidisciplinary group of health care professionals functions as several individuals with expertise in various areas working in serial fashion, separate from each other. Although overall objectives may be similar, they rarely work or meet together and even less frequently interact with the intent to overlap and interweave skill sets and care plans to arrive at those objectives. The multidisciplinary team is characterized by clear role definitions and consistent maintenance (even guarding) of the boundaries among those roles. A sports analogy would be a football or baseball team where each player has a specific position and assignment with only occasional deviation from these roles. Decision making and authority are centralized by design, and there is little, if any, tolerance, let alone permission, for innovation.

The interdisciplinary group may be composed of identical professional members as the multidisciplinary paradigm, but the role definitions are purposefully blurred and the boundaries are widely overlapping. Authority is shared, as is decision making, and innovation is encouraged wherever necessitated by patient need and circumstance. Referring to the previous sports analogy, the interdisciplinary group functions more like a basketball or soccer team where success results from fluid and spontaneous innovation, with some set plays but ample flexibility to adapt to the demands of changing situations. Roles are expected to be shared or traded as needed. In order to achieve this level of fluid teamwork, a high level of communication must be maintained which requires considerable maturity, trust, and intimacy. These professional expectations may exceed those required in other, less-interdependent health care environments.

Such teams or groups require an unusual degree of attention to interpersonal relationships in order to maintain the necessary level of mutual trust and understanding of one another's strengths and limitations. This need exposes the team to a significant risk, however. In order to achieve and sustain the ideal level of professional intimacy, it is often necessary to engage in a level of sharing that feels more personal than professional to the team members. As a result, team members may begin to look to the team to meet their personal needs and even to resolve issues in their personal lives. This is the one boundary a team must not cross. To do so runs the risk of undermining the team's professional functioning and blurs the focus of the team: delivering the highest quality of care possible to patients in need.

To maintain an optimum functional level, team members often must share and explore emotional reactions their patients and families trigger in them. However, this sort of sharing and self-examination should always be undertaken to further their professional functions, not as a means of meeting personal needs. Those must be met outside of the work environment in the intimacy of one's own personal life or in one's own decisions to partake of professional help in sorting through difficult emotional experiences.

A high functioning team must be flexible enough to reconfigure itself in response to the needs of each patient and family. This requires mature professionals who are able to deal with the personal and strong emotional issues hospice work engenders: one's own mortality, the motivations and sources that compel us to be a caretaker, one's need to be liked, ability to tolerate patients' anger, and so many others. While there can be intense and challenging issues, they should always and only be addressed in the effort to further the work at hand. We come together to asses and plan for the needs of our patients and families, not to address our own or our family's needs. The focus must always be the work: what serves the patient's and family's needs. The valuable time of team meetings needs to be spent addressing patient care issues first, then on personal issues as necessary in order to fulfill the care plan, and finally on interpersonal issues between or among team members when they become an impediment to care delivery. To depart from this healthy and functional approach is to depart from the reason the team exists.

The Structured Team Meeting

IDT Care Conference Format

This is a guide only, and it should be "molded" to fit the needs and unique circumstances of each team and the patients/families under care. Adherence to the *basic* format will ensure that most key issues are addressed and a focus on all pertinent elements is maintained. Keeping this format in mind during patient visits will also help to organize thinking and prioritize care issues.

Recommended IDT Conference Format for Patient Care Managers

- All disciplines represented and signed in
- Deaths reviewed since last IDT conference; lessons learned, thoughts and feelings about the care given and dying process
- New admissions (see "Two-minute" case presentation format later) home and other residential care (nursing home, long-term care, assisted living), inpatient settings
- Active problems (medical, psychosocial, practical, spiritual)
- Briefly review case load; indications for continuous care, inpatient admission (general inpatient and respite)
- Specifically review patients who will be due for recertification 2 to 3 weeks hence: address any questions regarding hospice eligibility, especially need for physician visit and "hands-on" reassessment
- A 15- to 20-minute mini "inservice" by team member(s) selected the previous week regarding a topic that emerged as "begging" deeper understanding and discussion by the team, or identified by patient care manager, such as symptom management, assessment/diagnosis, psychosocial issues, spiritual care issues, process/system (documentation, regulatory, compliance, etc.), bereavement
- Identification of topic and discussion leaders for next week's IDT conference "inservice"
- "Two-minute" case presentation by designated case manager, including patient name, age, gender, referring/primary physician, terminal diagnosis (*note: as much of this type of rostering that can be prepared in advance and automated, by using electronic media and projecting for the entire IDT to see, the better, because this will save time and reduce paper*), care situation (home, other); primary caregivers, current medications
  - Coexisting medical problems. Is there an adequate "database"? Is there a need for more information?
  - Interval history since last presentation
  - Symptoms well managed? Goals/needs met?
  - Continued problems, issues, needs, etc.
  - New problems, issues, needs, etc.
  - Progression of disease or level of debility (e.g., weight loss, decreased appetite, decreased energy/activity/function/ADLs, etc.); add specifics to documentation

- Review of determinants of limited prognosis for hospice admission diagnosis (supporting documents in medical record?)
- If symptoms are not well controlled, propose most likely etiology and specific treatment plan.
- Communication with referring physician: when, how, what?
- Is communication profile on referring physician complete? (i.e., profile of type of communication [telephone call, fax, email, letter] by whom and how often preferred by referring/primary care physician)
- Focused discussion led by patient care manager with input from IDT on the five "quality of life" domains as they pertain to the ongoing care of the patient/family under review:
  o Physical symptoms (pain, nausea, etc.)
  o Physical functions (activity, etc.)
  o Intrapersonal dimension (emotional status, self-view, etc.)
  o Interpersonal status (relationships, communication, conflicts, etc.)
  o Transcendant issues (issues of "meaning," existence, spiritual matters, etc.)
- In relation to the major end outcomes of end-of-life care:
  o Safe and comfortable dying
  o Self-determined life closure
  o Effective coping with loss and grief
- The plan of care should be derived from the above, including plan for communication with referring physician, delegation of duties to specific IDT members (who, what, when, how often, goals) and next scheduled review by IDT.

Addressing Needs Over Time

This section is meant as a guide for helping patients, families, and the caregiving team understand the dynamics of the last phase of life. Time frames represent generalizations that will need to be tailored to pertain to specific cases, but overall, they should help orchestrate care and prepare for the changes that tend to occur with advanced illness no matter where the patient resides.

Professional caregiver responsibilities, duties, and levels of involvement are assigned to those disciplines (core members of the IDT) that are most likely to have the greatest expertise in attending to the specified functions and needs of patients during the various phases of disease progression. These are not meant to be exclusive by any means. The true strength of the IDT is the ability of its core and additional members (e.g., pharmacists, nutritionists, functional restoration therapists), regardless of specific discipline, to fulfill multiple roles as the situation dictates, limited only by professional practice licensure restrictions and the experience and proven ability of the individual.

Hospice IDT Members: Approximately 6 Months or Longer Before Death

Patient and Family

- Patients are usually coherent and able to walk. They may have symptoms from previous medical treatments.
- Patient and family exhibit initial stages of grief with feelings of potential loss, anger, and denial.
- There may be humor and a heightened sense of living, all very appropriate.
- Some symptoms of decline (weight loss, fatigue) and a sense of the seriousness of the illness usually emerge.
- Initial signs of stress, with symptoms of depression, anxiety, or fear, should be anticipated and discussed.
- Family members wonder how they will cope.

Physician

- Reviews medical history; examines patient when indicated and certifies for hospice care
- Works with IDT to develop plan of care and authorizes medical orders
- Manages pain and other distressing symptoms
- Hospice physician attends interdisciplinary team meetings and confers with attending/referring physician as needed.

RN/Case Manager

- Communicates with physician, family, and patient to develop initial plan of care
- Ensures that medical orders and durable medical equipment are in place and trains/instructs nonprofessional caregivers
- Coordinates plan of care, providing direct patient care and directs other nurses, aides, and volunteers
- Manages resources
- Establishes rapport and trust with patient, family, and attending physician - Furthers discussions about advance care plans and end-of-life decisions
- Coordinates input at interdisciplinary team conferences.

CNA/HHA

- Initiates personal care program under direction of RN case manager
- Establishes rapport with patient and family and provides personal care
- Conferences with case manager in developing care instructions

Social Worker

- Elaborates hospice philosophy and services
- Assesses patient and family needs from a psychosocial and spiritual perspective
- Collaborates in development of a plan of care according to needs, goals, preferences, and hopes

- Provides support, problem-solving, coping strategies, and connections to other community resources as needed

Chaplain

- Collaborates with other team members as care plan is developed
- Meets with patient and/or family at their request for spiritual or related care
- Helps other team members providing psychosocial support and dealing with difficult issues

Volunteer

- Volunteer manager collaborates with interdisciplinary team to determine patient/family needs that may be fulfilled by volunteers.
- Arranges visits or telephone calls according to patient and family wishes and needs
- Assists with respite breaks and provides volunteer companionship when needed

Hospice IDT Members: A Few Months Before Death

Patient and Family

- Patient has decreased appetite, fatigue, and weight loss.
- Physical signs and symptoms are more evident. Family begins to reconcile feelings and plan for imminent death.
- Patient begins to accept the fact that disease is incurable and time is limited.
- Physical decline is apparent, and increased attention is spent on coping with progressive pain and other symptoms.
- Patient may show signs of social withdrawal, and the family may show signs of stress from caregiving and anticipatory grief.

Physician

- Works with IDT to evaluate symptoms, manage pain, and contribute to plan of care, adjusting medical orders as necessary
- Evaluates for continued hospice eligibility per guidelines

RN/Case Manager

- Monitors implementation of care plan with increasing attention to symptom management
- Assists IDT in evaluating and managing psychosocial needs

CNA/HHA

- Provides or assists in personal care as needed and directed
- Offers companionship
- Provides feedback to IDT about unmet needs and changes in status

Social Worker

- Monitors psychosocial plan of care and adapts it to changing needs and circumstances as they unfold
- Provides ongoing assessment of patient's and family's adjustment to the illness and impending loss and helps determine timing of respite based upon coping abilities
- Provides ongoing emotional support

Chaplain

- Provides spiritual and emotional support and counseling
- Communicates with clergy or lay spiritual leader of family/patient choosing
- Encourages and helps arrange rituals that offer meaning and support to the patient/family

Volunteer

- Works with volunteer coordinator, IDT, and patient/family to be aware of unspoken emotional or practical needs
- Spends "unstructured" time with patient and family in order to allow free exchange of concerns and feelings
- Helps relieve boredom for patient by engaging in whatever activities are feasible
- Works with IDT to identify ways and means to relieve caregiving burden

Hospice IDT Members: Last Few Weeks and Days
Patient and Family

- Symptoms tend to increase, with control of pain and shortness of breath chief symptom relief concerns.
- Fatigue becomes a dominant feature and the patient may be bedridden, requiring intensification of personal care and prevention of skin breakdown.
- The patient may alternately be extremely demanding and very withdrawn.
- Reinitiation of discussion regarding signs of imminent death, dealing with terminal care issues and funeral arrangements, is usually desired.

Physician

- Works with IDT to review symptoms with a focus on pain and other distressing symptom relief
- Contributes to biomedical aspects of the plan of care, adjusting medical orders as necessary
- Visits patient and family if symptoms are not readily controlled
- Available for rapid adjustment in medication orders and route of drug delivery as conditions dictate

RN/Case Manager

- Monitors patient closely, with increased frequency of home visits as dictated by changing conditions

- Frequent review of symptom control
- Coordinates care by members of IDT to support family and manage terminal care needs
- Determines whether continuous care or inpatient care is needed
- Instructs family in signs of imminent dying and to call so that attendance at death, or immediately thereafter, is possible

CNA/HHA

- Responds to changes in plan of care as directed by case manager
- Special attention to oral care, perineum, and pressure points
- Identifies special needs to IDT

Social Worker

- Anticipates and assesses for heightened anxiety and emotional distress, as well as caregiver fatigue
- Assists patient and family in resolving conflicts and making closure, expressing thoughts and feelings
- Helps family with funeral planning

Chaplain

- Continues to provide spiritual and emotional support
- Provides pastoral care as requested by the patient and family
- May assist with funeral arrangements and rituals
- Helps prepare family and patient for separation, and looks for ways to help heal relationships that are stressed, facilitating closure and the final opportunity for personal growth before death
- Familiarizes family with bereavement program, especially if bereavement counselor is a different person

Hospice IDT Members: After Death

- Family experiencing loss and grief

Physician

- May communicate with family; may send condolence note

RN/Case Manager

- Calls or visits family
- May attend funeral
- Assists bereavement counselor in assessing family's bereavement needs
- Completes documentation

CNA/HHA

- May attend funeral or visit family

Social Worker

- Calls or visits family
- May attend funeral
- Assesses family for signs of dysfunctional grieving and other psychosocial problems
- Makes referrals to appropriate resources

Chaplain/Bereavement

- May call or visit family
- May attend funeral
- Instructs family about grief recovery and support groups

Counselor

- Provides bereavement counseling as needed
- Plans and implements memorial services
- Directs staff and volunteers to maintain contact with family at regular intervals for 13 months

Volunteer

- May call or visit family
- May attend funeral
- Bereavement volunteers offer support for 13 months

Documentation

The Clinical Documentation Process Serves Several Important Functions

- It is the structure that describes what is to be done, what has been done, and what has been accomplished to meet the patient's/family's goals.
- It is the continuous and memorialized record of the patient and his or her experiences through hospice.
- Well-constructed records provide unambiguous and clear communication among all hospice care staff.
- The medical record is the means by which reimbursement for services is justified and determined.

Documents Must Serve the Needs of Many Different Persons and Organizations

Patient/Family

- Informative documents, brief and to the point
- As few signatures as possible
- Confidentiality
- Pertinent information only (respect for privacy, dignity, ethical boundaries) for delivery of quality care

Attending Physician and Referral Sources
- Brief, complete, summarized information
- Minimal paperwork burden

Interdisciplinary Team and Administrative Personnel
- Legible and timely entries
- Access to information
- Complete information
- Logical flow of information

Clinical Facilities (e.g., hospital, nursing home, inpatient unit)
- Facilitate continuity of care
- Logical flow of plan of care
- Summary information, encapsulated to provide brief but complete picture of the patient and other pertinent facts at time of admission

Regulatory Agencies, Third Party Payers, Accreditation Entities
- Proof of eligibility
- Zero tolerance for fraud/abuse of public funds
- Required for payment
- Critical step in regulatory compliance
- Complete entries
- Signed entries
- Adequate narrative to "tell the story" or "paint a picture" of the patient's/family's circumstances and experience through hospice
- Processes of care (evaluations, plans of care, interventions)
- Outcomes of care

Documentation and Risk Management

- Use full signature; date and time all entries.
- Complete all medical records and documentation forms (i.e., fill in the blanks).
- Be specific; elaborate only as necessary.
- Individual viewpoints are reviewed and reconciled at IDT conference, not in the written record. Discussions and challenge of ideas/perspectives are appropriate and welcome at IDT conference but have no place in the medical record.
- Report adverse occurrences/mistakes on incident reports.
- Legibility is key.
- Only use universally accepted abbreviations; when in doubt, spell it out.
- Read back verbal orders and note this confirmation to reduce medication errors.

Documentation Needs Specific to Hospice Care

- Routine home care: records must tell the story of the patient and reflect the patterns of care and the hospice experience.
- General inpatient care: records must clearly show the indications for a change in level of care.
  - Symptoms out of control
  - Efforts to regain control in the home
  - What interventions can be done in the inpatient setting that cannot be done at home?
  - Caregiver or environmental crisis needs to be well described.
  - If death is imminent, describe findings in detail.
  - Daily assessments, care plan, and IDT involvement need to be documented.
  - All interventions must be charted in detail, taking nothing for granted.
  - Specify what comfort measures were provided.
  - Must have frequent documentation, i.e., every 1 to 2 hours, not a synopsis; no "block charting," (e.g., 1–4 A.M.); charting must include specific times and events.
  - Document what the medical crisis was and continues to be that justifies this level of care.
- Initial certification and recertification: supply ample narrative that describes clinical parameters with respect to the hospice diagnosis and ongoing trajectory toward death.
- Define as clearly as possible "related" and "unrelated" conditions and therapies in relation to hospice diagnosis (e.g., diuretics are related to the diagnosis of end-stage heart failure, whereas insulin would be unrelated to this diagnosis).
- Utilize prognostic worksheets and guidelines and supplement with observations that support a prognosis of limited life expectancy.
  - o Track objective measures of decline (weight loss, reduced appetite, decreasing functional abilities, etc.).
  - o When decline is not apparent, describe care that may be leading to functional improvement and plans to review prognosis if improvement in status is sustained.
- Home health aide/certified nurse assistant supervisory visits: document supervision every 2 weeks—ensure compliance with state regulations.
- IDT Communication: comprehensive care plan updates are essential.
  - o Summarize communications in easy-to-review form
  - o Clearly state who (include discipline), what, when, why, anticipated goals, contingency plans, and next evaluation.
- Nursing home documentation: the record must show an integrated plan of care that clearly and specifically delineates hospice functions and identifies responsible staff:
  - o All care must be documented.

o Nursing home chart must have a specific place for hospice records.

o Medical orders must be duplicated and integrated into comprehensive plan of care.

Accountability

- All hospice staff are individually responsible and accountable for completing their respective portion(s) of the medical record in a legible and timely manner—this is a fundamental expectation and there are no exceptions.

- The RN case manager is chiefly responsible and accountable for coordinating care and assuring completeness of the medical records of the patients he or she is managing and, in turn, will monitor others' compliance. If deficiencies are not immediately corrected, the program director, or equivalent position, is to be notified so that corrective actions can be taken.

Section 2

Personal, Social, and Environmental Processes

Abuse in the Home

SITUATION: Domestic abuse or neglect interfering with end-of-life care

Findings

- Expression of ambivalent feelings of anger, jealousy, hurt, fear, sadness, guilt, self-righteousness, apologies, promises, or martyrdom
- Use of intimidation and manipulation as a way to maintain control and avoid feelings
- Family history of verbal, emotional, physical, economic, or sexual abuse
- Use of defense mechanisms: minimization, justification, denial, and blame
- Depression, suicidal ideation
- Physical evidence of abuse/neglect

Assessment

Physical

- Environmental or corporeal evidence of abuse, neglect, violence

Psychosocial

- Patient as victim of abuse
  o Identify patient/caregiver's perception of situation.
  o Assess history of abuse/neglect.
  o Assess patient fears.
  o Identify present threats of harm.
  o Identify if caregiver insists on staying close and speaking for patient.
  o Assess if patient is reluctant to speak or disagree in presence of caregiver.
  o Identify symptoms of depression, panic attacks, substance abuse, feelings of isolation, and post-traumatic stress reactions.
  o Determine patient/caregiver resources to address issue.
  o Determine support systems available.
  o Assess for risk of suicide.

- Patient as Abuser
  o Identify patient/caregiver's perception of situation.
  o Assess safety if patient is still physically capable of abuse.

- o Identify verbal and emotional abuse to caregiver by patient.
- o Assess need for control, manipulation, intimidation.
- o Assess presence of denial, minimization, justification, and blame as defense mechanisms.
- o Identify caregiver's ambivalent feelings/desire for revenge as barrier to provide adequate patient care.
- o Assess for intense emotional reaction to loss, including suicide potential.

Processes of Care

Psychosocial

- Patient as victim of abuse
  - o Facilitate discussion of perceptions and feelings.
  - o Acknowledge and encourage use of previously effective coping skills.
  - o Assist patient/caregiver in accepting limits imposed by illness.
  - o Assist patient/caregiver to develop new coping skills.
  - o Provide education on safety issues.
  - o See patient alone when possible.
  - o Visit with two staff members, one to see caregiver and one to see patient, to obtain clear information.
  - o Monitor willingness/ability to comply with treatment plan.
  - o Consider transfer to alternative location, e.g., care facility, if need arises.
  - o Confer with team members regarding intervention plan and options for care.

- Patient as Abuser
  - o Provide education on safety issues.
  - o Develop safety plan with team and caregiver.
  - o Assist in setting limits and clear communication about unacceptable behaviors with patient.
  - o Encourage patient to identify feelings underneath anger and need for control.
  - o Support caregiver in taking care of own needs.
  - o Provide additional support to give caregiver respite.
  - o Assist caregiver in making decisions on behalf of the patient that are not detrimental to caregiver.
  - o Discuss alternative with caregiver in situations of high risk/burnout, e.g., care facility placement.
  - o Confer with bereavement support staff regarding high risk for dysfunctional grief.

Goals/Outcomes

- Patient/caregiver will show improved ability to cope.
- Patient/caregiver/hospice staff will be aware of need for clear limits/boundaries for safety.

- Patient/caregiver will identify strategies to address needs in the terminal situation.
- Decreased incidence of domestic abuse/violence/neglect.

Documentation in the Medical Record

Initial and Ongoing Physical Assessment

- Examination findings suggestive of abuse, neglect

Initial and Ongoing Psychosocial Assessment

- Areas of abuse, neglect, and violence as identified by patient, family, and staff

Interdisciplinary Progress Notes and IDT Care Plan

- Specific interventions to assist patient/caregiver
- Patient/caregiver response to intervention
- Ongoing evaluation

Advance Care Planning and Directives for Healthcare Interventions

SITUATION: Patient has preferences about medical interventions and chooses to protect his/her rights by specifying the type of medical care desired.

State-specific advance directives can be obtained by accessing the NHPCO Caring Connections Website: http://www.caringinfo@nhpco.org.

Findings

- Patient wants to make decisions and protect his/her rights.
- Patient wants to clarify preferences to physician and caregiver/family.
- Family has differing ideas about treatment for patient.
- Patient wants to communicate choices while still able.

Assessment

Psychosocial

- Assess if advance directives have been previously completed.
- Assess patient/caregiver's awareness/understanding of value/purpose of advance directives.
- Assess patient's desire to complete forms with or without assistance from hospice staff.

Processes of Care

- *Psychosocial*

Educate patient and family about different types of advance directives and processes:

o Power of Attorney

Patient gives power to transact business on his/her behalf when he/she cannot do so because of time or distance (although physically able).

o Durable Power of Attorney

Patient gives power to transact business on his/her behalf when patient is no longer physically able.

o Living Will

This is an advance directive that states what types of care or medical interventions patient prefers or wishes to avoid under various circumstances.

o Durable Power of Attorney for Health Care

This legal document protects patient care choices by naming an advocate who makes decisions on behalf of patient when physician determines patient is not competent.

o Do Not (Attempt to) Resuscitate

This directive states that the patient refuses certain *potentially* life-prolonging medical interventions, such as cardiopulmonary resuscitation, chest compressions, endotracheal intubation, and defibrillation.

o Physicians Orders for Life-Sustaining Treatment (POLST)

Forms and educational programs intented to facilitate the greatest amount of patient self-determination in making end-of-life treatment decisions. This paradigm varies by state, with educational tools and forms for consumers and healthcare professionals. More information can be obtained by accessing the Website http://www.polst.org (accessed October 2006).

Guardianship

Parent is the guardian for minor child unless a legal action rules otherwise. Court appointed guardianship by petition can be temporary, financial, or custodial.

- o Facilitate discussion regarding choices for treatment/care with family when patient is no longer able to participate in these decisions.
- o Facilitate discussion with patient/caregiver regarding appropriate advance directives and choice of advocate.
- o Assist patient in completing advance directives form/document.
- o Procure a copy of advance directive for patient record.

Goals/Outcomes

- Patient will voice preferences about current and future medical care and actions to be taken in the event of loss of decision-making ability.
- Caregiver/family/advocate will have clear directions for understanding patient choices.
- Minimize ambiguity and ambivalence in all parties.
- Completion of life in a manner and setting consistent with wishes and values, i.e., "self-determined life closure."

Documentation in the Medical Record

Initial Psychosocial Assessment

- Need for advance directives as identified by patient/caregiver/social work/admission team
- Options discussed
- Forms/documents completed
- Copy of advance directives and documents in medical record

Interdisciplinary Progress Notes

- Documentation of processes of advance care planning that have been completed

IDT Care Plan

- Plan for carrying out processes of advance care planning

Changes in Body Image and Loss of Independence

SITUATION: Patient/caregiver reactions to changes in body image and loss of independence associated with advanced illness causing distress and difficulty coping/functioning

Findings

- Persistent, preoccupying, and intense expressions of anger, frustration, loneliness, loss of self-esteem, embarrassment, shame, guilt, etc. due to altered physical appearance, altered functional ability, changes in social/family identity/status
- Avoidance of discussion regarding appearance
- Loss of functional abilities due to disease process
- Increasing dependence upon others for care
- Caregiver loss of previously relied upon companion support; change in roles
- Social isolation
- Self-imposed disengagement from feelings, family members, friends, outside community
- Pronounced depression

- Sexual dysfunction
- Suicidal thoughts

Assessment

Physical

- Identify disease-related, postsurgical, or postradiation alterations in external physical features or means to communicate: e.g., amputation [including mastectomy; orchiectomy]; ostomies; open sores/wounds/lesions; scars or other disfigurement; vocal/visual/auditory impairment.

Psychosocial/Spiritual

- Identify primary issue(s) of concern.
- Explore patient/caregiver perception of body image, value of appearance, functional limitations.
- Determine patient/caregiver capacity to address the issues.
- Determine support systems available and nature/basis of faith/beliefs.
- Identify who patient will allow to help provide care .
- Assess for history of suicidal ideation or behavior.
- Rule out other confounding issues/comorbidities (e.g., depression, anxiety disorder, agoraphobia).
- Identify history/style of coping.
- Assess impact of illness/appearance upon sexuality.
- Assess financial resources available for supplementary help if needed.

Processes of Care

Physical

- Ensure that expert-level attention to wound and ostomy care, prosthetics, and other restorative or rehabilitative therapies, appropriate to the patient's overall circumstances, is arranged.

Psychosocial/Spiritual

- Facilitate expressions of feelings and perceptions; acknowledge losses.
- Address real versus perceived body image and functional limitations.
- Acknowledge and encourage use of previously effective coping skills.
- Provide information regarding progression of illness.
- Assist patient/caregiver to develop new coping skills for positive self-image.
- Encourage patient/caregiver participation in support groups.
- Treat identified mood disorder/phobic behavior with counseling.
- If symptoms are not responding to basic counseling approaches, assist in providing resources/referral to treat mood disorder/phobic behavior and support patient/family through crisis periods.
- Assist patient in finding meaning in past achievements through life review.

Practical

- Obtain consultation or access resources for use of prostheses, wigs, cosmetics, etc.
- Facilitate placement for respite and/or residential care if needed.

Biomedical

- Treat identified mood disorder with pharmacotherapy if indicated, per severity and diagnostic criteria.

Goals/Outcomes

- Condition-specific optimum physical and communicative capacities
- Patient/caregiver will demonstrate or verbalize improved coping ability.
- Patient/caregiver will express higher level of acceptance of alterations in body image and changes in functional abilities.
- Patient will exhibit less signs/symptoms of depression, anxiety, phobic behavior.
- Patient will feel less isolated.

Documentation in the Medical Record

Initial and Ongoing Physical Assessment

- Relevant physical findings and changes over time

Initial Psychosocial Assessment

- Evidence of poor body image/dependency and inadequate coping

Interdisciplinary Progress Note

- Manifestations of changes in body image and loss of independence
- Ongoing assessments and results of interventions

IDT Care Plan

- Defined interventions and expected outcomes

Changes in Family Dynamics

SITUATION: Family integrity and dynamics stressed so as to impact negatively upon effective end-of-life care

Findings

- Family member(s) report high level of stress due to inability to cope effectively with crisis of impending death and eventual loss of patient.
- Family member(s) exhibit difficulty with intimacy (dependency, conflict, or detachment).
- Family member(s) express concern/confusion about changes in roles, duties, lifestyle, and family interaction patterns.

- Family member(s) report other existing stressful issues requiring time and attention.

Assessment

Psychosocial/Spiritual

- Outline a "family tree" that describes the family system and defines roles, expectations, relationships, and issues.
- Identify family interaction patterns (e.g., close, conflicted, enmeshed, distant, or estranged).
- Ask family member(s) to describe their perception of family in the context of the patient's terminal illness.
- Identify previous experiences and patterns of dealing with loss individually and as a family system.
- Assess appearance of harmony or disharmony among various family members.
- Assess impact of conflicts on care of patient.
- Assess position the patient maintains within the family structure.
- Assess ability of family to communicate about dying.
- Assess existence of self-destructive/family-impacting behaviors (e.g., substance abuse, gambling or other addictive disorders) with any immediate family members including the patient.
- Assess history of mental illness, abuse, or antisocial behavior.
- Assess factors of illiteracy, or mental and physical limitations.
- Assess experiences and attitudes of family in dealing with the medical community or with authority figures.
- Assess willingness and ability to understand and utilize instructions and interventions.
- Assess impact of ethnic/cultural background, values, beliefs, attitudes, and family rituals/traditions.
- Assess ability of family system to access internal and external resources.

Processes of Care

Psychosocial/Spiritual

- Facilitate discussion of useful strengths and resources that successfully helped family member(s) in previous crises (e.g., cohesion, concern for each other, commitment to family, pride, loyalty, utilization of external resources).
- Increase awareness of family rules, boundaries, patterns of communication, and role expectations.
- Encourage dialogue and expressions of feelings about illness and dying, when appropriate.
- Identify role-change strain/conflict and assist in redistribution of roles and responsibilities.

- Assist family member(s) in setting short-, intermediate-. and long-term goals and acknowledge progress made in achieving them.
- Facilitate discussion of previous or ongoing hurt feelings that have potential for resolution/healing.
- Facilitate referral to external resources as needed.
- Facilitate arrangements for respite care, if appropriate, in family with high level of stress.
- Assist family in shared life review and reminiscence, if appropriate.
- Assist family in the task of preparing for the death of a family member.
- Assist family in the task of beginning to prepare for life after the death of the family member.
- Assist family in having realistic expectations of hospice care.
- Provide emotional support to family.
- Deal with resistance to psychosocial interventions.
- Develop plan of care with patient, family, and interdisciplinary team and continue to monitor progress.
- Facilitate family conference.

Goals/Outcomes

- Family shows increased ability to cope with the imminent death of a family member in the context of the family system.
- Family feels reduction in levels of stress.
- Family will have strengthened external/internal resources to care for patient at home, if this is the most appropriate setting.

Documentation in the Medical Record

Initial Psychosocial/Spiritual Assessment

- Dynamics of family system affecting care of terminally ill patient

Interdisciplinary Progress Note

- Summary of IDT conferences related to family dynamics impacting care
- Results of interventions
- Summary of ongoing evaluations

IDT Care Plan

- Resources and problem solving skills to be relayed/taught/recommended
- Social work interventions: who, what, when, how often, goals
- Chaplain interventions: who, what, when, how often, goals

Completing Worldly Business and Life Closure

SITUATION: Patient has a need to complete certain tasks before death.

Findings

- Patient expressing lack of completion in worldly affairs
- Patient/caregiver expressing desire for completion with relationships
- Patient expressing "weariness" with life; lack of purpose/meaning in living
- Patient/caregiver unable to accept patient's death
- Patient/caregiver unable to resolve spiritual issues
- Patient/caregiver working toward balance of body, mind, and spirit in the face of death

Assessment

Psychosocial/Spiritual

- Identify patient/caregiver perception of situation
- Identify patient/caregiver capacity to address life closure and/or unresolved issues
- Review past life experiences, changes in roles, losses, and previously effective coping skills
- Identify role-change strain/conflict
- Identify patient/caregiver experiences, concerns, and fears regarding the dying process
- Assess need for spiritual care and anticipatory grief support
- Assess patient/caregiver perception of current quality of life and future concerns

Processes of Care

Psychosocial/Spiritual—Worldly Affairs

- Support patient/caregiver in settling financial affairs and making final arrangements
- Link patient/caregiver with appropriate resources: financial/estate planner, viatical settlement organizations, legal counsel, etc
- Facilitate patient's writing of an estate will

Psychosocial/Spiritual—Meaning and Purpose in Life

- Assist patient in coming to terms with personal and existential loss represented by one's dying
- Facilitate patient/caregiver expressed need to search for meaning in the dying experience
- Review past life experiences, role changes, and losses

- Reinforce previously effective coping skills
- Help patient/caregiver search the meaning and depth of their particular faith/beliefs
- Assist patient in acceptance of dependence
- Refer to "complementary" therapies: music, art, massage, etc
- Assist patient toward growth/development in the context of personal grieving, loss, and suffering
- Relationships
  o Present grief as a unique opportunity to address and heal unresolved issues and fears
  o Facilitate closure with important relationships by expressing sorrow, forgiveness, affection, love, gratitude, appreciation, and saying "goodbye"
  o Assist patient in expressing self-worth and forgiveness
  o Involve caregiver in planning for emotional, spiritual, psychosocial, and physical needs and facilitate implementation
  o Facilitate discussion of useful strengths and resources that successfully helped family members in previous crises
  o Identify role-change strain/conflict and assist in redistribution of roles/responsibilities
  o Assist family in the task of preparing for the death of the patient
  o Facilitate and validate family rituals
  o Assist family in the task of beginning to prepare for life after the death of the patient
  o Refer, as appropriate, to grief support counselor for anticipatory grief

Psychosocial/Spiritual—Dying

- Respond to questions and concerns about the signs and symptoms indicating patient is approaching death
- Explore patient/caregiver experiences, concerns, and fears regarding dying process
- Support patient in letting go of worldly affairs and surrendering to the transcendent

Spiritual Issues

- Explore issues of guilt and human and/or divine forgiveness
- Encourage spiritual practices of meditation, keeping a written journal or audio/visual tape, imagery, prayers, and/or spiritual/religious rites
- Explore belief, faith, and trust in higher dimension that provide patient/caregiver support
- Assess need for spiritual care
- Respond to specific pastoral requests
- Encourage emotional/spiritual sharing among patient/family members

- Facilitate patient/caregiver connection with their preferred religious institution, if any

Goals/Outcomes

- Patient/caregiver will express increased sense of completion in worldly affairs
- Patient/caregiver will express increased sense of meaning and purpose
- Patient/caregiver to express increased sense of completion with relationships
- Patient/caregiver able to express acceptance of his/her death if possible
- Patient/caregiver to feel that there has been resolution of spiritual issues
- Patient/caregiver will have a sense of personal completion to life

Documentation in the Medical Record

Initial Psychosocial/Spiritual Assessment

- Major emotional, psychosocial, and spiritual issues of concern identified by patient, family, and hospice staff
- Coping skills, resources, preferences identified

Interdisciplinary Progress Note

- Continued identification of issues as per initial assessment
- Ongoing identification of goals
- Results and goals/outcomes summarized

IDT Care Plan

- Interventions planned by staff (who, what, when, frequency, goals)
- Plans for ongoing evaluation

Controlled Substances: Misuse and Abuse

SITUATION: Medically inappropriate use of controlled substances in the home negatively impacting end-of-life care

Findings

- Pattern of unexplained disappearance of medications
- Consistent shortage of prescribed controlled substance without appropriate communication to care team about medical necessity to change dose or schedule
- History or evidence of substance use among patient, family, and friends
- Deliberate guarding or expression of need to guard medications from others
- Environmental clues that suggest drug diversion
- Unusual patient or family perceptions of symptom management

Assessment

Psychosocial/Spiritual

- Identify substance abuse as reported by patient/caregiver and/or observed by professional care team member(s)
- Identify characteristics of chemically dependent family system as evidenced by the following patterns:
  o Denial
  o Control
  o Conflict
  o Distrust
  o Unresolved losses
  o Secrets
  o Resistance to outsiders
  o Blaming
  o Domestic chaos
  o Violence
  o Falsification
- Identify prior or current use of formal treatment and support programs (i.e., AA, NA, ALANON, NARANON, etc.).
- Understand patient and family perceptions regarding symptom management and substance abuse.
- Assess impact of substance use on ability to provide patient care or to cope with dying.
- Refer to the *Diagnostic Statistical Manual, Fourth Edition (DSM-IV)* in completing assessment.
- Assess need to intervene and/or refer to specialty counseling or mental health services based on impact of substance abuse.
- Understand special social/cultural/ethnic/religious perspectives (rituals) of patient/caregiver/family member(s) on controlled substance use.

Processes of Care

Educational

- Provide information regarding effects of substance abuse on physical symptoms and grief processes.
- Provide information and instruction regarding achievable expectations regarding symptom management.

Psychosocial/Spiritual

- Explore motivations for substance use (abuse), especially if a new problem.
  o Depression/despair/hopelessness
  o Anxiety
  o Fear
  o Anticipated grief
  o Other conflicts

- Involve family in talking about options and interventions.
- Use appropriate referral sources.
- Develop unified team approach.

Practical/Procedural

- Schedule II/III medicines (e.g., opioids, benzodiazapines) are to be reordered by only one nurse.
- Renew only 1-week supply at a time.
- Count medication carefully each nursing visit.

Goals/Outcomes

- Patient/caregiver will verbalize understanding of appropriate medical use of prescription medications for symptom management (schedule and dose).
- Patient/family will utilize outside resources for specific issues related to substance abuse as necessary to attain patient end-of-life goals.
- Effect(s) of substance abuse on patient care or ability to cope will be minimized.

Documentation in the Medical Record

Initial Psychosocial/Spiritual Assessment

- Explicit findings of substance abuse
- Current and projected impact on patient/caregiver/family

Interdisciplinary Progress Note

- Interventions carried out (who, what, when)
- Expected goals/outcomes
- Results of interventions
- Findings of ongoing evaluations and assessments

IDT Care Plan

- Schedule of interventions
- Contingency plans if interventions do not achieve hoped-for outcomes
- Schedule of follow-up and reevaluations
- Changes in care plan with justification

Cultural Differences: Respect, Understanding, Adapting Care

Note: The citizenry of the United States is ethnically, religiously, and racially diverse. This brief overview is meant to serve as both a reminder and a guide so that professional caregivers can meet the varied needs of individuals within our culturally heterogeneous society.

SITUATION: The patient/family under care has significantly different values and customs than the professional caregivers.

Findings: Initial and ongoing patient/family assessment will reveal a wide range of cultural differences, such as

- Country of origin, sense of nationality, ethnic background
- Language, dress, interpersonal behavior and interpretation of caregivers' spoken and "body" language (e.g., eye contact, "personal space," manners/mannerisms, etc.)
- Attitudes toward individuality, autonomy, self-determination, and place within the family and society
- Attitudes toward illness, dependency, dying, and death
- Attitudes toward food, meals, and nutrition
- Attitudes toward pain and suffering
- Attitudes toward modesty and gender roles
- Expression of spirituality: religion/religious institution, faith, rituals, beliefs

Assessment, Processes of Care, Goals/Outcomes, Documentation

In order to provide meaningful end-of-life care, a thorough understanding of the patient's/family's cultural imperatives and values is necessary. This may be particularly challenging when there are language barriers, so every reasonable attempt should be made to obtain capable translation. If at all possible, caregivers or volunteers should be assigned who have some experience with the particular cultural values system of the patient/family, and the IDT can then be better educated to the particular nuances that will affect care.

The entire hospice team needs to be committed to providing assistance without prejudice to all people with limited life expectancy who want our help. This mission demands the highest regard for individual rights and freedoms in accordance with the laws of the land. Due to the diversity of people in our society, it is more likely than not that we will encounter individuals who are very different from ourselves. In order to be true to the principle of patient-centered and family-focused care, insight into the values of those who invite us into this phase of their lives is a necessity. Only through conscious attempts at understanding can unintended bias and unwitting "cultural blunders" be prevented.

It is beyond the scope of this manual to elaborate all the various cultural differences that exist toward dying and death. Nevertheless, the hospice professional is encouraged to expand her/his knowledge with an open-minded and inquisitive attitude whenever the opportunity presents itself. There are many resources for learning in every community: church groups, cultural organizations, local libraries, and the Internet, among other sources, can provide helpful background. And, under most circumstances, patients and families are extremely pleased that someone is interested in seeing the world through their eyes. Most important, your willingness to understand and appreciate others' life views in the midst of their coming to terms with life and death will be valued beyond measure.

Denial

SITUATION: Problematic expressions of denial that interfere with attainment of patient-directed goals, care of patient, ability to cope

Findings

- Family insists that patient not be told prognosis.
- Resistance to accepting available support and help to the extent that inadequate care is rendered and patient goals are not able to be realistically assessed/attained
- Preoccupation with somatic symptoms with a view toward rediagnosis/cure in the face of appropriate diagnostic/prognostic information given
- Inability to acknowledge patient's physical and/or mental decline
- Excessive resistance to planning for future without patient
- Excessive resistance to talk about prognosis
- Patient/family making unrealistic future plans

Assessment

Psychosocial/Spiritual

- Explore and understand patient and caregiver's perception of situation.
- Explore and understand motivations for (purposes served by) denial.
- Assess history of coping style with prior losses.
- Assess impact of denial on family dynamics, symptom management, safety issues, and ability to cope.
- Review and understand beliefs/faith and support systems of patient/caregiver/family.

Processes of Care

Practical

- Educate caregiver/family and care team about denial as a usual and healthy coping strategy, and the potential for maladaptive denial to interfere with good care and the attainment of goals.

Psychosocial/Spiritual

- Approach denial openly, thoroughly supporting it as a constructive self-protective coping mechanism.
- As appropriate, assist patient, caregiver, and family to confront the issues of denial and develop plans to achieve relief of unresolved concerns.
- Assist patient/caregiver to develop alternate constructive coping strategies as situation dictates.

Goals/Outcomes
- Patient/caregiver will address denial as barrier to patient care
- Maladaptive coping styles will decrease at least to the extent that adequate assessment of realistic and potentially attainable goals and care can take place
- Patient/caregiver will more productively understand/utilize denial as an adjustment mechanism and as a response to loss to enhance remaining time before death
- Patient/caregiver will make progress toward making final plans and funeral arrangements

Documentation in the Medical Record
Initial Psychosocial/Spiritual Assessment
- Degree to which denial is playing a role in coping
- Evidence of maladaptive denial: interference with ability to adequately evaluate goals, expectations, hopes, etc.; interference with ability to ensure basic safety and/or quality care
- Risk for lack of closure and/or pathological grief

Interdisciplinary Progress Note
- Ongoing area(s) of denial
- Interventions and outcomes

IDT Care Plan
- Schedule of interventions: who, what, when
- Contingency plans if first set of approaches not beneficial
- Schedule of follow-up and reevaluation: who, when

Grief Reactions

SITUATION: Excessive grief interfering with patient/caregiver ability to function or cope
Findings
- Excessive sadness, anger, guilt, anxiety, loneliness, fatigue, hopelessness, numbness (lack of attachment, dissociation), helplessness
- Sleep disturbance
- Eating disturbance
- Social withdrawal
- Restless or frenetic activity/compulsive or repetitive behaviors
- Somatic preoccupation, symptoms
- Mood disturbance (depression, mania)

- Impulsive behaviors
- Functional impairment
- Suicidal ideation
- Onset or exacerbation of addictive behaviors, including eating, smoking, alcohol abuse, gambling

Assessment

Psychosocial/Spiritual

- Identify cultural background, traditions, and attitudes regarding death/grief
- Understand spiritual beliefs/religious affiliation and practices
- Understand how family expresses emotions
- Define realistic parameters of life-expectancy/prognosis
- Determine the patient's role in the family and the potential impact of the loss
- Review prior history of previous experiences with loss and coping style/skills
- Assess suicide potential/ideation
- Assess support systems
- Assess substance abuse, if indicated

Biomedical

- Evaluate sleep patterns, eating patterns, mood, functional limitations, suicidal risk.

Interdisciplinary Team

- IDT to review, compare, and consolidate findings in order to determine the degree to which anticipatory grief is maladaptive and harmful

Processes of Care

Psychosocial/Spiritual

- Provide information on the grieving process
- Encourage patient/caregiver to talk about his/her losses
- Involve family in problem solving/goal setting
- Assist patient/caregiver to identify and express emotions
- Reinforce positive coping strategies
- Suggest and help develop new or more adaptive coping strategies
- Reinforce benefit of caregiver involvement in directly caring for patient and acknowledge/validate these efforts
- Encourage participation in physical and social activities
- Encourage expressive activities such as writing, painting, music, crafts, gardening, etc
- Elicit preferences and help facilitate family rituals

- Mobilize bereavement support resources including extended family, friends, community groups, religious organization or other spiritual care when valued by patient/caregiver/family
- Facilitate funeral planning with patient/caregiver
- Slowly and carefully assist caregiver to explore ways to restructure life without patient
- Identify complicated and pathological grief reactions and refer to appropriate mental health resource
- Encourage participation in grief support programs
- Consult with bereavement support staff

Biomedical

- Treat disordered mood and sleep with appropriate medications on a short-term basis if not rapidly responsive to nonpharmacological approaches

Goals/Outcomes

- Patient/caregiver will verbalize understanding of normal grief response
- Caregiver will utilize grief support services as appropriate
- Patient/caregiver will express emotions related to grief
- Patient/caregiver will verbalize sense of increased ability to cope with grief
- Extreme and pathological grief reactions will be identified early so that appropriate resources can be mobilized

Documentation in the Medical Record

Initial Psychosocial/Spiritual Assessment

- Grief reactions manifested by patient/caregiver.

Interdisciplinary Progress Note

- Ongoing observations and evaluation of grief reactions
- Results of specific interventions

IDT Care Plan

- Specific interventions: who, what, when, how often
- Contingencies for poor response to primary interventions

NOTE: Processes of grief and bereavement in children are developmental age dependent (see Table 2.1). Anticipated and aberrant reactions must be readily distinguished and specially trained (pediatric) staff must intercede quickly when unhealthy behaviors are evident.

Table 2.1 Grief and Bereavement in Children

BIRTH TO SIX MONTHS

Characteristics of Age	View of Death and Response	What Helps
• Basic needs must be met, cries if needs are not met • Needs emotional and physical closeness of a consistent caregiver • Derives identity from caregiver • View of caregiver as source of comfort and all needs fulfillment	• Has no concept of death • Experiences death ike any other separation—no sense of "finality" • Nonspecific expressions of distress (crying) • Reacts to loss of caregiver • Reacts to caregiver's distress	• Progressively disengage child from primary caregiver if possible • Introduce a new primary caregiver • Nurturing, comforting • Anticipate physical and emotional needs and provide them • Maintain routines

SIX MONTHS TO TWO YEARS

• Begins to individuate • Remembers face of others, caregiver when absent • Demonstrates full range of emotions, feelings and interactions • Identifies caregiver as source of good • No control over feelings and responses; anticipate regressive behavior	• May see death as reversible • Experiences bona fide grief significant • Grief response only to death of significant person in child's life • Screams, panics, withdraws, becomes disinterested in food, toys, activities • Reacts in concert with distress experienced by caregiver	• Needs continual support, comfort • Avoid separation from close physical and emotional connections • Maintain daily structure and schedule • Support caregiver to reduce distress and maintain a stable environment Acknowledge sadness that loved one will not return—offer comfort

TWO YEARS TO FIVE YEARS

• Egocentric • Cause-effect not understood • Developing conscience • Developing trust • Attributes life to objects • Feelings expressed mostly by behaviors • Can recall events from past	• Sees death like sleep: reversible • Believes in magical causes • Has sense of loss • Curiosity, questioning • Anticipate regression, clinging • Aggressive behavior common • Worries about who will care for them	• Remind that loved one will not return • Give realistic information, answer questions • Involve in "farewell" ceremonies • Help put words to feelings; provide ways to remember loved one • Keep home environment structured, stable • Encourage questions, expression of feelings • Reassure child who will take care of them

FIVE TO NINE YEARS

Characteristics of Age	View of Death and Response	What Helps
• Attributes life to things that move; may fear the dark. • Begins to develop intellect • Begins to relate cause and effect; understands consequences • Literal, concrete, may feel responsible • Decreasing fantasy life, increasing control of feelings	• Personifies death as ghosts, "bogeyman" • Interest in biological aspects of life and death • Begins to see death as irreversible • May see death as punishment; needs strong parent • Problems concentrating on tasks; may deny or hide feelings, vulnerability	• Give clear and realistic information • Include child in funeral ceremonies if they choose • Give permission to express feelings and provide opportunities; reduce guilt by providing factual information • Maintain structured schedule, individual and family activities • Notify school of what is occurring, gentle confirmation, reassurance

PREADOLESCENT THROUGH TEENS

Characteristics of Age	View of Death and Response	What Helps
• Individuation outside home • Identifies with peer group; needs family attachment • Understands life processes; can verbalize feelings • Physical maturation	• Views death as permanent • Sense of own mortality; sense of the future • Strong emotional reactions; may regress, revert to fantasy • May somaticize, intellectualize, morbid preoccupation	• Unambiguous information • Provide opportunities to express self, feelings; encourage outside relationships with mentors • Provide tangible means to remember loved one; encourage self-expression, verbal and nonverbal • Dispel fears about physical concerns; educate about maturation; provide outlets for energy and strong feelings (recreation, sports, etc.); needs mentoring and direction

Living Environment, Finances, and Support Systems

SITUATION: Inadequacy of living environment, finances, or support systems that interferes with patient care or ability of patient/caregiver to cope with illness/dying

Findings

- No caregiver or frail or otherwise limited caregiver
- Insufficient food, heat, electrical power, protection from extremes of weather
- Infestation
- Hazards, e.g., faulty wiring, heating, waste disposal/sanitation, or structures; unsecured weapons (guns, rifles, ammunition)
- Dangerous behaviors (e.g., smoking with oxygen or unattended while in bed)
- Isolation, e.g., inadequate transportation/telephone or inability to communicate due to language barrier or other communication problem
- Insufficient financial resources for basic needs or expenses associated with illness and dying
- Ongoing or imminent legal matters, disputes

Assessment

Psychosocial/Practical

- Assess physical environment, and understand social support systems and extent of resources.
- Identify legal decision-makers for patient.
- Understand needs and wants of patient/caregiver; desire to change.
- Define barriers to improving compromised situation.
- Define financial and practical needs: food, shelter, heating/cooling, phone, transportation, funeral and burial expenses, uncovered medical expenses, legal expenses.
- Determine unrealized sources of federal, state, and community assistance.
- Help to determine current and future expense, income, and assets.

Processes of Care

Psychosocial/Practical

- Address environmental concerns with patient/caregiver.
- Develop action plan among team to help make environmental improvements as acceptable to patient (utilize volunteers and community resource networks).
- Provide home safety education and plan.
- If safety and other basic concerns cannot be corrected, facilitate placement in a more secure environment if acceptable.

- Determine extent to which patient/caregiver will accept volunteers, home health aide, continuous care, and respite care to provide needed support.
- Provide information and help to procure financial assistance and social services; assist with application processes, and serve as liaison/facilitator/advocate with institutions and agencies.
- Offer help with budgeting.

Basic Home Safety

Environment
- Electrical safety: risk of electrical shock or fire
  - o Remove electrical cords from beneath carpet and rugs.
  - o Recommend replacement of worn, cracked, spliced, frayed electrical cords.
  - o Reduce extension cord and multiple outlet adaptor overload.
- Floor safety: risk of falls and injury
  - o Remove or secure loose rugs, runners, mats with appropriate fixation (tacks, adhesives, rubberized matting).
  - o Secure loose carpet edges.
  - o Recommend repair of uneven walkways or damaged flooring.
- Outside communication: help in case of emergency
  - o If at all possible, place telephone where it is most accessible most of the time.
  - o Emergency telephone numbers should be posted on or near telephone in large bold print.

- Fire safety
  - o Recommend one smoke detector on every level of home.
  - o Develop evacuation plan or review existing one with patient/caregiver; assign specific roles to capable live-in family members in case of fire.
  - o Establish clear pathways to all exits.
  - o Have key(s) accessible near key-locked (deadbolt) doors.
  - o Inquire if actively used chimneys have been inspected; recommend annual inspection.
  - o Kerosene heaters, wood stoves, and fireplaces should not be left unattended while in use.
- Bathroom safety
  - o Tubs and showers should have nonskid surface/mats to prevent slips and falls.
  - o Grab bars to assist transfers should be installed in tub, shower, and toilet area as needed.
  - o Adjust hot water heater temperature to avoid hot water burns; check water temperature on sensitive body part before bathing/showering (patients with sensory neuropathy are particularly vulnerable).
  - o Use nightlights in the bathroom and hallways en route to bathroom.

- Bed safety
  - Assess need for pressure sore prevention and bed rails, and obtain safe/effective equipment as indicated.
- Stairs and passageway safety
  - Stairs, hallways, and passageways between rooms should be well lit and free of clutter.
  - Stairs should have sturdy, well-secured handrails on both sides.
  - Avoid using stairs while wearing only socks or smooth-soled shoes/slippers.
- Outdoors
  - Entrance ways should be clear of leaves, snow, and ice.
  - Recommend and assist with making arrangements to clear entryways in snowy weather.

Medical Supplies

General

- Storage: keep supplies in a cool, dry, clean area protected from children and pets.
- Handling: make sure patient/caregiver has been given proper instruction on use and handling of all medical supplies and equipment, especially avoidance of injury and contamination.
- Disposal: instruct patient/caregiver that all dressing materials and disposable equipment that has been in patient contact should be wrapped in newspaper, bagged and placed in a completely secure trash area.

Oxygen

- Storage: oxygen and tubing should be kept away from open flames or heat sources.
- Handling: should be handled only by people who have been properly instructed by nursing personnel or medical equipment representatives.
- Disposal: used tubing should be disposed of in the manner described above; all other equipment should only be removed by professional personnel.

Drugs

- Storage: cool, dry place, secure from children and pets.
  - Determine the best balance between safety and convenience for the patient/caregiver.
  - Determine whether medications require special handling or refrigeration. Review expiration dates.
- Handling: ensure that all medications are adequately labeled.
  - Check name, dose, and time schedule before giving/taking any medication.
  - Observe patient taking medications to determine independent capability.
  - Give instruction for refilling prescriptions on a schedule prior to using up current medication supply.

- o Count medication doses on a regular basis for those prescriptions to be taken on an "around the clock" schedule to ensure appropriate utilization.
- Disposal: old, unused, or discontinued controlled substances, should be flushed down the toilet.
  - o Chemotherapy drugs must be returned to the hospital for disposal.
  - o When in doubt, speak to pharmacy.

Needles and Syringes ("Sharps")

- Storage: cool, dry place, secure from children and pets
- Handling: examine for signs of contamination before opening.
  - o All caregivers and patient need to be instructed in proper use, protection, and disposal.
  - o Observe caregiver/patient capability prior to independent use.
- Disposal: place used "sharps" in supplied puncture-resistant container to be returned to the hospice office for disposal.

Infectious Waste

- Storage: do not store.
- Handling: use gloves, confine to patient area, secure all materials in double plastic bags.
- Disposal: flush all excretions/secretions down the toilet.
  - o Dispose of contaminated materials as described above.
  - o Cleanse reuseable containers by soaking in a 1:10 dilution of household bleach for at least 30 minutes.

Parenteral and Enteral Solutions

- Storage
  - o Store unopened enteral solutions/mixes at room temperature and administer at room temperature.
  - o Opened cans or mixes for enteral feeding must be covered, dated and timed, and refrigerated and should be used within 24 hours of opening.
  - o Parenteral solutions should be stored in a refrigerator (except lipids) and removed 1 hour prior to administration.
  - o Parenteral solutions should be infused within 24 hours.
- Handling
  - o Use clean technique when handling enteral solutions.
  - o Use aseptic technique when handling parenteral solutions.
- Disposal: dispose of all unused, partially used or expired materials consistent with local ordinances and conventions. As environmental standards within communities become updated, an annual call to the state health department environmental office is recommended in order to maintain compliant policies and procedures.

Goals/Outcomes

- Develop a safe and comfortable environment for patient/caregiver and hospice staff.
- Appropriate use of medical equipment, supplies, and medications
- Decrease financial and legal worries concerning patient care issues.
- Maintain patient/caregiver preferences and dignity as much as possible, balanced against safe working conditions for professional/volunteer staff.

Documentation in the Medical Record

Initial Psychosocial/Practical Assessment

- Environmental assessment, risks, barriers to care
- Determination of support systems
- Definition of financial and legal issues that may impact care

Interdisciplinary Progress Notes

- Instruction in basic safety measures (environmental, medical)
- Summation of discussions regarding options for environmental, financial, legal help and patient/caregiver responses, preferences
- Description of interventions
- Results of interventions

IDT Care Plan

- Description of interventions: who, what, when
- Contingency and follow-up plans and alternatives based upon results of discussions/interventions and patient/caregiver response

Suicide: Risk, Prevention, Coping If It Happens

SITUATION: Patient expressing thoughts or wishes for self-inflicted/assisted death or suicide occurs

Findings

- Signs and symptoms of severe depression
- Overwhelming sense of hopelessness, meaninglessness, purposelessness, despair
- Expression of death wishes
- Devaluation of life and living
- Suicidal ideation, gestures, plan
- Sense of giving up and giving in (blissful euphoric affect or despair)
- Repeated expressions of being a burden, excessive guilt or shame
- Feelings of being abandoned (by friends, family, God)

- Accrual of large doses of central nervous system–depressant drugs (opioids, hypnotics, sedatives, anxiolytics, etc.)
- Prior history of major depression, impulsive behavior, suicide attempt(s)

Assessment

Biomedical

- Determine whether any physical symptoms are out of control and patient/caregiver beliefs, perceptions about symptom control issues
- Review medications and determine if symptoms may reflect drug-related adverse effect.

Psychosocial/Spiritual

- Review prior history of depression, anxiety, absence of coping skills, and suicide attempt(s) and formally assess for signs and symptoms of major depression (refer to the *DSM-IV*).
- Review coexisting social/environmental stresses that may be contributing to sense of despair (separation/divorce, loss of job, income, prestige, etc.).
- Evaluate family/caregiver behaviors that suggest patient is burdensome.
- Evaluate beliefs/faith and understand patient's value system (self-view, sense of hope and hopelessness, meaning, purpose, etc.).
- Understand patient's expressed wishes to end life if able to articulate them.
- Determine if there is a concrete suicide plan.
- Determine high risk of imminent suicide by presence of:
   o Specific suicide plan
   o Availability of resources to carry out plan
   o History of prior suicide attempts
   o Misuse of medications/alcohol
   o Hearing voices to kill self
   o Inadequate social support
   o Agitation or flat affect coupled with despair

Processes of Care

Biomedical

- Vigorously treat all out-of-control symptoms.
- Initiate antidepressant therapy if indicated and monitor closely.

Psychosocial/Spiritual

- Low risk: no plan, no substantial ideation, no significant risk factors
   o Assist in identifying positive aspects of patient's life and areas of "unfinished business."
   o Help to establish attainable short-term goals.
   o Assist in developing and strengthening relationships.

- o Address issues regarding self-image and any distorted thinking.
- o Provide 24-hour contact and consider continuous care if suicidal ideation increases.
- o Offer pastoral care or facilitate involvement with existing spiritual/religious leader.
- o Invite discussions regarding sense of meaning and purpose.
- o Assist in providing activities to assuage boredom.
- o Involve family/caregiver in discussions with patient regarding sense of burden.
- o Help to arrange respite for family/caregiver as necessary.
- o Educate entire IDT as to level of risk and need to monitor for increased risk.
- Moderate to high risk (substantial ideation and plan with significant risk factors, per above)
  - o Utilize interventions as described above.
  - o Notify physician.
  - o Explain limits of professional confidentiality applied to potential suicide.
  - o Discuss negative consequences of suicide.
  - o Attempt to establish a verbal or written "no suicide contract."
  - o Instruct caregiver to observe for changes in mood or behavior and who to notify.
  - o Attempt to remove all lethal agents.
  - o Provide multiple contacts (crisis line, suicide prevention, hospice, chaplaincy).
  - o Daily visits from patient-preferred hospice staff member who has expertise in suicide prevention and management of depression and adjustment reactions.
  - o Arrange mental health expert consultation as needed.
- Occurrence of suicide
  - o Notify physician for appropriate completion of death certificate.
  - o Provide intensive bereavement support and counseling to family/caregiver.
  - o Refer family/caregiver to support groups as needed and per family preference.
  - o Provide "debriefing" and staff support for IDT members intimately involved in care.

Goals/Outcomes

- Enable patient's sense of purpose and meaning in remaining existence.
- Prevent suicide without stripping patient of dignity, autonomy, and rights of self-determination.
- Attain closure and functional grieving for family/caregiver and staff if suicide occurs.

Documentation in the Medical Record

Initial Biomedical Assessment

- Formal evaluation for symptom control and severe mood disorder

Initial Psychosocial/Spiritual Assessment

- Define level of risk and options discussed.
- Document contributing factors.

Interdisciplinary Team Notes

- Results of discussions, reassessments, and specific interventions
- Documentation of suicide prevention plan and change in level of risk

IDT Care Plan

- Specific interventions and contingency plans (who, what, when)
- Follow-up plan

Section 3

Clinical Processes and Symptom Management

Pain and symptom management is a key focus of hospice care, because it is rare for people who are experiencing severe physical distress to consider other aspects of their existence. Improvements in pharmaceuticals and pharmacotherapy have served to enhance the ability to keep distressing symptoms associated with advanced disease under reasonable control in the vast majority of cases. Therefore, excellence in pharmacotherapy plays a critical role in the provision of high-quality hospice care, so solid grounding in this area is the starting point for the hospice clinician's knowledge base. A fundamental principle is that all medication management must be tailored to the individual needs and situation of the patient. The information provided in this section is meant to guide therapy and should not be used rigidly in lieu of clinical judgment. Pharmacoeconomics always plays a role in current-day health care, so cost considerations will enter into decision-making at some level. These analyses should be used in order to make balanced decisions after sound assessment principles have been followed, leading to an indication for a therapeutic intervention.

Knowledgeable clinicians recognize that many symptoms (e.g., pain, anxiety, restlessness) have an oftentimes lengthy differential diagnosis. For example, restlessness may reflect metabolic encephalopathy, air hunger (dyspnea), hypoxia, pain that is poorly localized or difficult to express, social stress, an unresolved emotional or spiritual issue, and so forth. Furthermore, each of these etiologies has its own lengthy differential diagnosis that may require further evaluation and specific treatment.

It is always incumbent on the clinician to make the best determination of the CAUSE of the distressing symptom in order to promote the best PALLIATION of the symptom. The more closely these are matched, the more likely it is that the patient's (and caregiver's) needs will be met. With this in mind, pharmacotherapy may not always be the best approach to symptom management. When it is, this guide should serve as a means of making this process more uniform and timely, actualizing the goals of maximizing therapeutic effect and minimizing adverse effects. Careful titration of drugs, especially when using polypharmacy (more than one drug at a time), is required to avoid toxic effects, especially when drug-drug interactions and synergistic effects are likely to occur. These should be understood, anticipated, prevented, and monitored. The effects of aging amplify many drug effects, and these principles and precautions should be accentuated in older individuals.

Because many symptom and treatment domains are overlapping (e.g., dysphagia and painful mucositis) cross- referencing will serve to make this resource as useful and compact as possible. When issues are not crystal clear, we can and should rely on the strength, diversity, and breadth of experience within the interdisciplinary team to find direction. True emergencies (e.g., pain out of control, extreme agitation, severe dyspnea) should trigger immediate intervention and, when necessary, consultation. For medically oriented problems, this guide should serve as a reference for immediate action, to relieve suffering as quickly as possible.

Clinicians should always choose the drug formulation that is believed to best serve the patient's needs, after all pertinent variables have been considered. Although clinical experience is invaluable, reliance on anecdotal experience alone is a dangerous trap. Generally speaking, extemporaneous formulations (compounding) should be avoided in favor of commercial formulations, becaue the latter are subject to considerable regulatory scrutiny and quality control, so factors such as dissolution and absorption are far more likely to be predictable. Last, expense is always a consideration in health care, and hospice in particular, due to its payment structure under the Medicare Hospice Benefit. Cost-effective therapies should drive clinical decision-making, not cost containment. Good business practices combined with skilled case management should allow all patients to obtain the most beneficial treatments available in order to optimize therapeutic outcomes.

Air Hunger (Dyspnea)

SITUATION: Shortness of breath, chest tightness, air-hunger often associated with findings of anxiety, panic, desperation, or impending doom

This symptom is often more distressing than pain. Although it is very important to formulate a differential diagnosis as quickly as possible in order to match treatment with the identified cause whenever possible, **never delay palliative treatment for any reason**. *Air hunger is probably the most terrifying symptom that can be experienced, and panic can overcome even the most stable and well-prepared patient, family, and other caregivers. THE EMERGENT TREATMENT OF CHOICE (unless a cause is immediately identified that can be treated just as readily and quickly) IS MORPHINE (OR AN EQUIVALENT IF THERE IS MORPHINE ALLERGY/SENSITIVITY). THE MOST RAPID AND MOST READILY ACCESSIBLE AND IMMEDIATELY AVAILABLE ROUTE OF ADMINISTRATION SHOULD BE USED. Choices include the following:*

- Oral morphine concentrate (20 mg/ml): 1/4 to 1/2 ml sublingual (SL)/oral (PO); repeat in 10 to 15 minutes as needed
- Nebulized morphine (parenteral grade, preservative free) 2.5 mg in 2 to 4 ml 0.9% (normal) saline or fentanyl 25 to 50 µg (1/2 to 1 ml) in the same volume of saline is an alternative if preferred by the patient

- Parenteral opioid delivery via the subcutaneous (SQ) route is feasible in most settings

  For patients who have established intravenous access, it may be preferable and faster to titrate intravenous morphine, starting with 1 mg every few minutes in opioid-naïve patients, or an equivalent opioid (e.g., 10 μg fentanyl; 0.15 mg hydromorphone)

  The dose of opioid, regardless of route of administration, should be adjusted based on previous experience and opioid tolerance of the patient.

Causes

Practical

- Excessive or poorly regulated activity (pacing issues)
- Improper physical positioning (e.g., orthopnea)

Psychosocial Psychosocial/Spiritual

- Anxiety associated with dyspnea itself—i.e., a vicious cycle—or anxiety from other sources of worry, angst, etc., serving as a trigger for dyspnea
- Fear (usually compounded by experiences from previous episodes)

Biomedical

- Pulmonary disease (e.g., chronic obstructive pulmonary disease [COPD], restrictive lung disease, pneumonia)
- Pleural effusion
- Pericardial effusion
- Neuromuscular disease affecting coordinated mechanics of breathing and respiratory muscle function
- Uncompensated heart failure
- Weakness, fatigue, aesthenia due to primary disease or secondary causes (e.g., metabolic derangement, myesthenia)
- Anemia with inadequate oxygen carrying capacity
- Acute pulmonary embolism (PE)
- Acute myocardial infarction (MI)

Findings

- Anxiety, restlessness, fearfulness, agitation, "panic facies"
- Complaint of shortness of breath or similar expression of breathing difficulties
- Inability to speak in complete sentences due to running out of breath
- Decreased functional ability due to shortness of breath
- Increased use of accessory muscles of respiration and posturing to catch breath (head forward, pursed lip breathing, sitting bolt upright)
- Tachypnea
- Cyanosis, hypoxemia

Assessment

Practical

- Air circulation
- Dust, pollen, pet hair, strong perfumes/cleansers, etc.
- Patient positioning, availability of pillows, bolsters, etc.
- Proximity of medications, caregiver
- Knowledge and understanding of crisis prevention plan

Biomedical

- Review diagnosis and likely medical etiologies for symptoms.
- Vital signs (respiratory rate, pattern, depth; pulse rate and quality; blood pressure [BP]; temperature)
- Cardiac examination: rate, rhythm, peripheral perfusion, venous distention
- Pulmonary examination: quality of breath sounds (wheezes, rales, rhonchi/rattles, acute changes)
- Extremity examination: edema, skin turgor, pallor
- Abdominal examination: acute distention, ascites, tenderness
- Check oxygen saturation (portable pulse oximeter) for acute changes
- Patient self-rating of intensity/severity of episode(s) using a standardized numerical (0 to 10) scale (verbal or visual, depending on patient preference and capability) with 0 being "no shortness of breath" and 10 being "worst shortness of breath imaginable." Repeat measurements should be taken and noted after intervention(s); Link patient/caregiver self-care and crisis prevention/intervention plan to severity ratings after some experience with this type of tool
- Occasionally, laboratory evaluation of hemoglobin/hematocrit to determine potential causes of limited oxygen-carrying capacity may be necessary if first-line palliative measures are not proving to be effective

Psychosocial/Spiritual

- Acquire history of previous experiences, interventions, worries, plan for preventing crises, and potential emotional triggering factors

Processes of Care

Practical

- Avoid gas-forming foods to prevent gastric/bowel distention
- Discuss and facilitate remedial environmental adjustments to decrease symptom triggers and improve respiratory mechanics (e.g., rest periods, pacing, raise head of bed, use of bolsters, etc.)
- Instruct patient/caregiver in optimum patient positioning, day and night
- Provide durable medical equipment (DME) as needed for positioning
- Provide air movement using a fan and/or humidifier if at all possible and determine symptomatic utility

- Teach percussion and vibration to caregiver(s) as indicated
- Devise crisis prevention and care plan
- Review regularly: what to do, when and who to call
- Check patient/caregiver understanding
- Optimize accessibility and availability of prophylactic/therapeutic/communication resources

Biomedical

- Notify physician if any unexpected or significant changes in physical examination that may require change in care plan or physician evaluation
- Institute oxygen therapy ONLY if demonstrated that patient is hypoxemic AND there is a therapeutic response to the use of supplemental oxygen. Otherwise, use personal fans or other means of increasing air circulation
- Optimize medical management (diuretics, vasodilators, bronchodilators)
- Consider trial of passive positive pressure (external) breathing device, if available
- Palliative pharmacotherapy
  o Primarily anxiety-triggered dyspnea:
  o Anxiolytic therapy: lorazapam PO/SL/SQ 0.5 to 2 mg q2-4hr or PRN
  o Primarily non-anxiety-triggered dyspnea:
  o Opioid therapy: rapidity of onset and therapeutic effect is a function of establishing blood levels as quickly as possible
  o For patients with intravenous access, titrate IV doses to effect q5-10min (e.g., morphine sulfate 1 mg or equivalent) to determine patient's sensitivity and threshold for response
  o For patients without intravenous access, similar SQ doses can be given, or administer oral morphine concentrate (20 mg/ml) titrated to effect, starting with 0.25 to 0.5 ml SL/PO. Alternatively, nebulized morphine 2.5 mg in 2 to 4 ml 0.9% (normal) saline or fentanyl 25 to 50 µg in the same volume of saline is recommended. The medical literature is inconclusive about this form of therapy, but anecdotal experience has been favorable in some patients, especially as an alternative to establishing intravenous access or much slower absorption routes (SQ/SL). This symptom should be anticipated in susceptible patients so that the apparatus for nebulizer treatments is readily available
  o An alternative to nebulized or parenteral drug delivery in order to establish rapid patient-controlled levels of opioid is oral transmucosal fentanyl citrate (OTFC). A 100-200 µg dose provides opioid tolerant patients a noninvasive, self-administered means of relieving dyspnea for those without IV access, SQ dosing, or immediate access to nebulizer set-up. There is limited clinical experience with this technique

NOTE: Titrate dose slowly to effect, especially when using in combination with opioids, to determine patient's sensitivity.

o Continued therapy with opioid analgesics by the most convenient route with an anxiolytic (lorazapam PO/SL/SQ 0.5 to 2 mg q2-4hr or PRN) is usually necessary until death unless there is a well-defined remediable cause (see later)

Treatable Causes

1. Bronchospasm: A history of asthma or COPD is usually present. Listen for expiratory wheezes. Use a nebulized β_2-agonist (e.g., albuterol). Inhaled corticosteroids (e.g., beclomethasone) are proving to be beneficial in relieving acute bronchospasm. Systemic corticosteroids (e.g., prednisone) may be required in refractory cases.

2. Pulmonary edema: Volume overload and left ventricular failure, leading to right ventricular failure, are the most common causes. Restriction of fluids and limiting sodium intake (or artificial feedings) and use of morphine therapy may relieve acute symptoms. In refractory cases, consider initiating or advancing diuretic therapy (furosemide 40 to 240 mg), inotropic therapy (digoxin), and angiotensin-converting enzyme inhibitor (ACE) therapy, according to clinical signs and symptoms, assessed by auscultation of heart and lungs, jugular venous distention, peripheral edema, and balance of fluid intake and (urinary) output.

   In severe cases, where urgent palliation is indicated, parenteral diuretic and opioid drug administration is warranted, by the most convenient route (IV, IM).

3. Bronchial obstruction by tumor: Consider radiation therapy if prognosis allows; corticosteroid therapy for end-stage palliation, e.g., dexamethasone up to 12 mg/day in divided doses; and for symptomatic relief, nebulized fentanyl and lidocaine have also been used with varying degrees of efficacy.

4. Pleural effusion: Consider thoracentesis only if symptoms are not readily managed by noninvasive means (opioid and benzodiazapine pharmacotherapy, positioning, diuretics) and there is likelihood of significant improvement in performance status or return to a level of functioning meaningful to the patient. In the final days of life, thoracentesis (especially if not able to be performed in the home) adds a greater burden than benefit. If nonloculated peripheral pleural effusions recur within days, and the relief of symptoms was viewed as meaningful to the patient, consideration for pleurodesis is appropriate in patients with a life expectancy of more than a few weeks.

5. Superior vena cava syndrome (obstruction of the SVC): dexamethasone 24 mg IV followed by aggressive symptom control with corticosteroid, opioid, and benzodiazapine pharmacotherapy while considering the merits of radiation therapy (for patients with an otherwise predicted life expectancy of more than a few weeks).

6. Ascites: Diuretic therapy (e.g., furosemide 40 mg PO and spironolactone 100 mg PO day, titrated upward as needed to maximum daily doses of furosemide 240 mg, spironolactone 400 mg) is the first line of therapy. However, diuretics are rarely helpful in cases of malignant ascites. In termi-

nal disease states, paracentesis is rarely indicated. In cases of slowly developing ascites leading to dyspnea, where the burdens of symptom-relieving pharmacotherapy (opioids plus benzodiazapines) seem to outweigh the benefits, paracentesis should be considered if there is a life expectancy of several days to weeks.

7. Secretory conditions: Consider scopolamine SQ (0.2 to 0.4 mg) or transdermal; or glycopyrrolate 0.2 mg SQ and saline nebulizer treatments.

Psychosocial

- Teach relaxation techniques, cognitive-behavioral techniques, and breathing exercises
- Address worries and fears in a direct, supportive way; help problem-solve when concrete issues arise
- Reduce anxiety by assuring patient and caregiver that measures to improve symptoms will be taken immediately

Goals/Outcomes

- Reduced frequency and intensity of dyspneic episodes, with concurrent decrease in distress
- Improved sleep, appetite (if applicable), social interaction, mood, interest in what life has to offer
- Improved functional status (if applicable), e.g., self-care, time out of bed, toileting out of bed, etc.
- Decreased work of breathing
- Elimination of crises and unwanted interventions and transfers (e.g., ambulance calls, hospitalizations, intubation, etc.)

Documentation in the Medical Record

Initial Medical Assessment

- Pertinent systemic review, examination findings, diagnostic impressions
- Dyspnea rating (patient self-report)

Initial Practical/Psychosocial/Spiritual Assessment

- Nonmedical initiating and contributing factors

Interdisciplinary Progress Notes

- Results of interventions
- Changes in biomedical, psychosocial, spiritual issues and circumstances influencing symptoms and management
- Repeat dyspnea ratings (patient self-report)

IDT Care Plan

- Nonpharmacological and pharmacological interventions with appropriate medical orders

- Follow-up and contingency plans
- Crisis prevention/intervention plan

Agitation and Anxiety

SITUATION: Anxiety or agitation that is distressing to the patient/caregiver or negatively impacts on care of the patient or the caregiving environment

Severe anxiety (or panic) and uncontrolled agitation represent some of the few, but true, emergency conditions (along with severe dyspnea and pain) in the hospice setting. Anticipation and early recognition of these circumstances with a prevention and treatment plan are critical to optimum care of the dying.

Causes

Biomedical

- Respiratory distress (e.g., dyspnea from any cause; symptomatic hyoxemia and/or hypercarbia)
- Uncontrolled pain
- Primary anxiety/panic disorder
- Disease-induced psychosis (e.g., brain metastasis, metabolic disturbance)
- Drug-related psychosis (e.g., corticosteroids)
- Sleep deprivation
- Agitated depression
- Full bladder, fecal impaction, nausea in a patient who cannot otherwise express distress other than through behavioral response
- Substance abuse/misuse/withdrawal (e.g., alcohol, opioid, benzodiazapine abstinence syndrome)

Psychosocial/Spiritual

- Response to imminent loss (anticipatory grief)
- Fear of the unknown and other fears associated with severe illness and imminent death
- Nightmares/night terrors

Findings

- Verbal or other expressions of anxiety, panic, terror, fear, worry
- Disordered sleep
- Misuse of prescribed medications and noncompliance with other treatment protocols
- Abusive language or behaviors toward caregivers
- Push of speech, tangential thoughts, perseveration
- Volatile behavior; combative behavior

- Altered appetite
- Somatization
- "Panic" behaviors (e.g., frequent impulsive telephone calls, dialing 911)
- Increased complaints of pain that are not responsive to analgesic medication management
- Autonomic nervous system reactions (tachycardia, diaphoresis, tachypnea)
- Sense of impending doom or death without accompanying biomedical signs

NOTE: *In advanced disease states, especially cancer, differentiating physical symptoms due to anxiety from those attributable to somatic, visceral or neurogenic manifestations of the disease may be extremely difficult. Empirical therapy may be required.*

Evaluation

Biomedical

- Evaluate for concomitant evidence suggesting an organic brain syndrome due to advancing disease with either local or systemic manifestations (e.g., hallucinations, nausea/vomiting, papilledema, hypo/hyperglycemia, uremia).

NOTE: *Laboratory testing should only be done if findings will specifically alter or influence the plan of care to alleviate distressing symptoms.*

- Review medications for adverse drug reactions (e.g., psychotropic drugs, analgesics, corticosteroids).
- Ensure that all medications whose abrupt discontinuation can lead to an acute abstinence syndrome are either maintained or slowly tapered.

NOTE: *Consult with physician or pharmacist for dosage conversion and formulations if an alternative route of administration is necessary.*

- Conduct systems review and examination of bladder and bowel function (e.g., urinary retention, constipation, impaction).
- Examine less-than-fully coherent or noncommunicative patients for signs of unrecognized pain source (e.g., bone pain, abdominal pain, decubitus pain, etc.).
- Respiratory examination for potential cause of hypoxemia/dyspnea (respiratory rate and pattern, use of accessory muscles, pallor/cyanosis, rales, pleual effusion, etc.)
- Cardiac examination for evidence of heart failure, ischemia or arrhythmia (rate, rhythm, jugular venous distention, peripheral/pulmonary edema, diaphoresis)

Psychosocial/Spiritual

- Patient self-rating on anxiety scale (if capable)
- Caregiver rating of patient on agitation scale
- Assess patient/caregiver perceptions of cause/source of anxiety/agitation.
- Review past experiences with significant losses and deaths.

- Review current and past history of anxiety/panic disorder and psychiatric care; refer to *Diagnostic Statistical Manual, Fourth Edition (DSM-IV)* for diagnostic criteria.
- Identify coping skills/social support and barriers to care.
- Observe interactions among caregiver(s)/patient.
- Assess impact of anxiety/agitation on overall care.
- Identify areas of unresolved conflict.

Processes of Care

Biomedical

- If hypoxemia-induced agitation responds to a trial of oxygen therapy, maintain oxygen administration protocol with usual recommendations and precautions.
- Attempt to reduce dyspnea by increasing air circulation with a portable fan.
- Listening-talking therapy should precede or supplement pharmacotherapy unless symptoms are immediately uncontrollable or at crisis levels.
- Nightmares or terrifying hallucinations and severe anxiety or agitation should be controlled emergently for the patient's and family's sake.

Pharmacotherapy for acute and recurrent anxiety

1. Lorazapam 0.5 mg PO/SL/SQ q2-4hr. Titrate dose and interval as needed. Oral formulations of lorazepam (PO/SL) are considerably less costly than parenteral formulations. Sublingual lorazepam has been shown to be absorbed (attain plasma levels) similarly to parenteral administration.
2. In a crisis, without intravenous access, deep IM injection of lorazepam (1 to 2 mg) or diazepam (5 to 10 mg) is the most expedient means to attain a calm setting in which to seek out more specific treatment approaches (complete the assessment) or institute longer-term maintenance therapy.
3. Patients who are not responsive to low-moderate dose benzodiazepine therapy require further evaluation.

Pharmacotherapy for acute and recurrent agitation

1. Mild-moderate restlessness or delirium: haloperidol 0.5 to 5 mg PO/IV q4-6hr (titrate upward as needed) or chlorpromazine 10 mg IV or 25 mg PO/PR q6-8hr (titrate upward as needed).
2. More severe delirium and terminal restlessness (involuntary movements) often require more rapid dose titration and combination therapy. Paradoxical reactions to sedative drugs can occur. These effects should be recognized quickly so that alternative therapies can be instituted.
   a. Start with above-noted therapies (lorazepam plus haloperidol or chlorpromazine). Add nembutal suppository 60 to 120 mg PR q4hr as needed. Diphenhydramine 25 to 50 mg PO/IV q6hr should be used if extrapyramidal effects are noted when using haloperidol or chlorpromazine (avoid these drugs in patients with Parkinson's disease).

b. An expensive but effective alternative for control of terminal agitation symptoms poorly responsive to first-line therapies above is SQ infusion of midazolam: subcutaneous bolus dose of 5 mg followed by 1 mg/hr. Titrate up or down according to level of consciousness and emergence of symptoms.

c. Another costly but effective treatment for total sedation in an inpatient setting is propofol infusion. This requires a functional intravenous line and the supervision of a clinician experienced in the management of total sedation utilizing this technique. Usual doses for initiating therapy are 10 mg (1 ml) incremental boluses in rapid succession (q1-5min, depending on patient's circulation time) until effective sedation versus respiratory function is achieved. Continuous infusion at a rate of 10 to 50 μg/kg/hr is usually the effective range, but this must be titrated to individual circumstances and response. Propofol can be painful when infused through a peripheral vein. The addition of preservative-free lidocaine in a ratio of 40 mg lidocaine: 200 mg propofol (1 ml 4% lidocaine added to each 20 ml propofol) is effective in eliminating pain during bolus or infusion.

Psychosocial/Spiritual

- Teach relaxation, imaging, and distraction techniques when applicable.
- Openly discuss feelings, perceptions, role changes, losses, and issues of control and frustration.
- Interact with patient/caregiver in a calm, reassuring manner.
- Use life review and story-telling techniques to engage patient and discern sources of conflict.
- Acknowledge and reduce fears and worries by providing information and clarifying distortions in thinking in a gentle and sensitive manner:
  o What can the patient/caregiver expect over the next days to weeks?
  o What is usual course of the disease and prognosis?
- Be open and invite all questions; look for the meaning behind "cloaked" questions.
- Reinforce coping skills and anxiety-reducing behaviors/techniques.
- Facilitate problem solving and decision making.
- Provide instruction on how to create a calm environment for patient and caregiver (be aware that paradoxical effects may occur—some people prefer chaos):
  o Reduce noise, bright light, clutter
  o Increase structure, schedules, orderliness
- Design crisis intervention plan for emergency management of out-of-control symptoms.
- Have pharmacotherapy orders available (see above under "Biomedical").
- Have hospice on-call telephone number immediately available.

- Hospice staff to consult with physician if symptoms do not respond to interventions within reasonable time period (1 to 4 hours, depending on severity of symptoms)

Goals/Outcomes

- Episodes of anxiety/agitation will be reduced in frequency and intensity in order to reduce both distress to the patient and caregiver burden.
- To provide an opportunity for reconciling internal and interpersonal conflicts
- To eliminate the likelihood of self-harm or injury to caregivers
- To prevent avoidable transfers and discontinuity in care setting whenever possible

Documentation in the Medical Record

Initial Psychosocial/Spiritual Assessment

- Anxiety Score recorded using standard analog scale (patient report)
- Agitation Score recorded using standard analog scale (caregiver report)
- Manifestations of anxiety/agitation
- Ability of caregiver to cope with patient's condition
- Social/environmental factors that contribute to anxiety/agitation

Initial Medical Assessment

- Medical findings and contributors to anxiety/agitation
- Physical manifestations of anxiety/agitation
- Effects of anxiety/agitation on medical condition
- Current medication and other substance use for pain, insomnia, restlessness, anxiety/agitation

Interdisciplinary Progress Notes

- Anxiety Score recorded using 0-to-10 scale (patient report)
- Agitation Score recorded using 0-to-10 scale (caregiver report)
- Patient/caregiver response to proposed interventions (e.g., agreement, denial, defensiveness, disregard, anger, etc.)
- Patient/caregiver compliance/acceptance of care plan
- Results of interventions and reassessments

IDT Care Plan

- Proposed interventions: who, when, what
- Contingency plans and reassessment schedule
- Crisis prevention/intervention plan

Anorexia and Cachexia

SITUATION: Progressive decline in appetite, nutritional status, and body mass as a result of catabolic changes associated with chronic disease

Findings

- Decreased or no appetite with lack of interest in eating
- Feeling of fullness after minimal ingestion of food (early satiety) that may result from organomegaly ("squashed stomach")
- Continuous underlying presence of nausea
- Changes in taste perception, often unpleasant
- Dehydration, uremia, hypercalcemia, and other metabolic alterations
- Oral candidiasis, mucositis
- Gastritis

Evaluation

Practical

- Environmental assessment to determine source(s) of unpleasant odors
- Determine food preferences, reactions to various foods (what is particularly pleasant/unpleasant) and recent food intake, patterns of hunger/eating if any, and practical limitations such as ability to chew, swallow, use of dentures, etc
- Determine patient/caregiver understanding and capability to prepare modified foods (e.g., blended, pureed), if there are barriers to obtaining foods (e.g., transportation, finances), and any practical limitations of food storage or preparation (e.g., refrigeration, cooking, infestation)

Biomedical

- Identify underlying causes or contributing factors that may be subject to palliation, correction, or treatment if the patient's sense of well-being is negatively impacted by signs/symptoms.
  - o Pain
  - o Nausea
  - o Uremia, hypercalcemia
  - o Constipation, obstipation, impaction
  - o Bowel obstruction
  - o Hepatomegaly
  - o Depression
  - o Oral candidiasis
  - o Mucositis, esophagitis, gastritis
  - o Xerostomia (dry mouth)
- Assess patient's ability to swallow

- Assess symbolic value of nutrition/hydration to patient/caregiver (nurturing, guilt) and identify areas of patient/caregiver conflicting opinions, beliefs, or values related to feeding/hydration
- Determine to what degree anorexia/cachexia signs and symptoms are disturbing to patient/caregiver and what preferences/goals/concerns exist about these

Processes of Care

Practical

Facilitate means to reduce environmental factors that negatively influence patient interest/enjoyment in meals and suggest enhancements such as:

- Preprandial alcoholic beverage of choice, if acceptable and tolerated
- Effort made to take meals in esthetically pleasing environment with companionship rather than in bed or sleeping area
- Have patient suck on hard candy (trial and error of sweet versus sour/citrus) to mask bad tastes.
- Involve patient in menu planning.
- Try very small portions with more frequent feedings, if patient is interested.
- Suggest cold (semi-frozen) nutritional drinks to overcome difficulties with chewing, swallowing, and odor/taste aberrations if patient is interested.

Biomedical

- Inform patient/caregiver of relative risks/burdens versus benefits of various routes of alimentation and hydration as applicable.
- Palliative pharmacotherapy (in order of demonstrated efficacy):

  1. Corticosteroids
     a. Dexamethasone 1 to 2 mg PO tid
     b. Methylprednisolone 1 to 2 mg PO bid
     c. Prednisone 5 mg PO tid
  2. Hormonal therapy
     a. Megestrol acetate 80 to 160 mg PO qid
  3. Other approaches
     a. Dronabinol 2.5 mg PO bid to tid
     b. Cyproheptadine 8 mg PO tid
     c. Thalidomide has been found to reduce anorexia/cachexia associated with HIV disease, although it is very costly compared with other available medications.

Psychosocial/Spiritual

- Reassure patient/caregiver/family that anorexia/cachexia are usual occurrences associated with progressive chronic diseases.
- Help open up discussion regarding any conflicts that may exist concerning nutrition and hydration.

- Educate and dispel myths about utility of alimentation (enteral or parenteral) under conditions of "wasting" diseases.
- Discuss ethical/moral concerns regarding alimentation and hydration in the face of life-limiting illness.

Goals/Outcomes

- Amount, frequency, and type of alimentation/hydration will be commensurate with attainable preferences/goals of patient and appropriate to disease state.
- Decrease symptoms attributing to or associated with anorexia/cachexia that are disturbing to patient.

Documentation in the Medical Record

Initial Practical/Psychosocial/Spiritual Assessment

- Findings related to environmental factors contributing to troublesome symptoms
- Elaboration of issues pertaining to preferences, goals, and values related to alimentation/hydration; copy and place specific advance directives in chart

Initial Medical Assessment

- Review of systems and history pertaining to and associated with anorexia/cachexia
- Physical findings, stage of disease, nutritional status

Interdisciplinary Progress Notes

- Description of interventions
- Results of interventions
- Ongoing evaluation of mental and physical status

IDT Care Plan

- Goals/outcomes
- Timing of interventions, visits, and contingency plans
- Medical orders for pharmacotherapy

Belching and Burping (Eructation)

SITUATION: Distress or discomfort associated with frequent belching or persistent gastric distention

Causes

Biomedical

- Aerophagia (air swallowing; may be secondary to anxiety)
- Indigestion

- Gastroparesis, ileus, or small bowel obstruction
- Excessive oral secretions or difficulty managing secretions
- Dysfunctional swallowing (cranial nerve or motor impairment)

Psychosocial

- Anxiety

Findings

Biomedical

- Feeling of epigastric or substernal fullness/pressure; excessive pressure may refer pain to chest or cause esophageal reflux with symptoms of "heartburn"
- Nausea/vomiting
- Abdominal distention (tympany; diminished or excessive bowel sounds [borborygmas])
- Oral lesions and/or excessive secretions
- Impaired swallowing

Psychosocial

- Anxiety state
- Embarrassment
- Social isolation

Evaluation

Biomedical

- Review nutritional status and food intake as cause of excessive gas production.
- Assess and rule out bowel dysmotility.
- Examine oropharynx, cranial nerves, and swallowing action.

Psychosocial

- Patient self-rating on anxiety scale (if capable)
- Caregiver rating of patient on agitation scale
- Determine the degree of distress symptoms are causing patient and family; this will help determine how aggressively symptom management should be approached
- Assess patient/caregiver perceptions of cause/source of anxiety/agitation if these emotional factors are believed to be contributory
- Identify coping skills/social support and barriers to care
- Observe interactions among caregiver(s)/patient
- Assess impact of symptoms on overall ability to meet other care goals

Processes of Care

Biomedical

- Evidence of bowel obstruction or ileus should be immediately brought to the attention of the physician before instituting any other therapy
- Mild to moderate symptoms may be reduced by using carbonated beverages to induce air elimination (best to try in presence of staff so that results can be evaluated; discontinue immediately if symptoms worsen)
- Adjust positioning in bed to elevate head to at least 30 degrees
- Dietary instruction to avoid foods that cause indigestion or are difficult to chew and swallow; encourage smaller, more frequent meals
- Instruct patient to thoroughly chew simethicone tablets, if able
- Pharmacotherapy
  1. Simethicone 80 mg chewable tablets before every meal and at HS as needed
  2. For anxiety-related symptoms, refer to Section Three—Agitation and Anxiety.
  3. For oropharyngeal problems, refer to Section Three - Dysphagia and Oropharyngeal Problems

Psychosocial

- Teach relaxation, imaging, and distraction techniques when applicable
- Reinforce coping skills and anxiety-reducing behaviors/techniques

Goals/Outcomes

- Relief of distention and excessive belching
- Reduce physical and psychological distress

Documentation in the Medical Record

Initial Medical and Psychosocial Assessment

- Potential cause(s) of eructation
- Physical examination findings (cranial nerves, swallowing, oropharynx, abdomen)
- Amount of distress/discomfort caused by symptoms
- Remedies tried by patient/caregiver with degree of success

Interdisciplinary Progress Notes

- Results of selected interventions and ongoing assessments

IDT Care Plan

- Interventions and contingency plans

Bleeding, Oozing, and Malodorous Lesions

SITUATIONS:

- Bleeding: minor, moderate, or major bleeding leading to distress, fatigue (anemia), excessive caregiver burden
- Malodorous lesions, exudates, drainage, etc.: these problems represent sources of great social distress for patients and their caregivers. Even the most loving family members and caregivers may find it difficult to stay in close contact with the patient when smells from infected or necrotic tissues and the like can be so overwhelming. Similarly, patients will feel humiliated, undignified, and isolated, feeling "unlovable." This type of situation most flagrantly adds insult to injury, and all that can be done should be done to diminish the burden of sensory insults that drive a wedge between patient and caregivers/loved ones.

Causes

- Necrotic tissue due to tumor or ischemia
- Erosion of vascular supply by tumor
- Breakdown in skin integrity
- Infection
- Gastrointestinal disease: gastritis, peptic ulcers, inflammatory bowel disease, tumor, varices
- Nonhealing wounds due to inadequate blood supply or catabolic state
- Bleeding diathesis/coagulopathy

Findings

Biomedical

- Malodorous and oozing lesions, drainage sites
- Minor bleeding:
  - o Minor recurrent nosebleeds (epistaxis) or gingival bleeding caused by drying of mucous membranes or increased systolic blood pressure
  - o Capillary oozing or other minor bleeding from open sores, decubiti, stomas, hemorrhoids, macerated/abraded skin (e.g., perineum)
- Moderate to major bleeding:
  - o Gastrointestinal blood loss (melena, hematochezia, hematemesis)
  - o Pulmonary blood loss (hemoptysis)
  - o More vigorous blood loss from epistaxis, skin lesions, stomas, etc., as above
- Disruption of major blood vessel(s) by necrosis or tumor
- Fatigue, dyspnea, tachycardia, hypotension
- Pain may be associated with bleeding, oozing, infected, necrotic lesions
- Nausea, vomiting, diarrhea may be associated with swallowed blood or gastrointestinal bleeding

Psychosocial/Spiritual

- Fear
- Disgust
- Isolation
- Avoidance
- Depression
- Anxiety
- Panic

Evaluation

Biomedical

- Determine source and cause of unpleasant bodily odors and drainage.
- Minor bleeding:
  o Determine source of bleeding.
  o Inspect open wounds and dressings for evidence of bloody drainage.
  o Determine rate/amount of bleeding.
  o Examine to identify specific bleeding site, if possible.
- Moderate to major bleeding:
  o Determine likelihood of massive hemorrhagic (exsanguinating) bleed
  o Determine site, cause, and volume of active blood loss, if possible.
- Determine relationship between signs and symptoms of fatigue with degree of anemia induced by blood loss.

  NOTE: Only check hematocrit if infusion of blood products is an appropriate palliative measure in the whole context of the patient's circumstances, preferences, and goals and if bleeding site has been controlled adequately to prevent immediate loss of transfused red cells.

- Determine caregiver knowledge and ability to manage wound care and dressing changes.

Psychosocial/Spiritual

- Assess emotional effect of malodorous or oozing lesions and bleeding on patient/caregiver.
- Review or initiate discussions regarding advance directives in the face of massive blood loss.
- Identify any specific injunctions against the use of blood products.

Practical

- Identify readily accessible resources to deal with massive blood loss (e.g., dark towels, etc.).

Biomedical

- Malodorous and oozing lesions: The primary approach to wound care is cleansing with sterile saline. Use of peroxide or iodine-containing solutions should be reserved for cases where there is infection or necrotic tissue so that granulation is not inhibited. Necrotic tissue may require active debridement, progressing from wet-to-dry dressings, to Xerogel or similar dressings, to application of enzymatic agents (e.g., streptokinase).
- Management of malodorous lesions includes:
  1. Cleansing with dilute sodium hypochlorite, hydrogen peroxide, povidone-iodine, or chlorhexidine solution, as tolerated.
  2. Application of an outer layer of charcoal dressing to absorb odor, where practical
  3. Use of metronidazole
     a. Topical 0.75% gel
     b. Systemic use, if tolerated, 500 mg PO tid
- Painful cutaneous lesions (see Section Three - Pain)
  1. NSAIDs are often helpful; e.g., ibuprofen 10 mg/kg PO tid (maximum 2400 mg/day)
  2. Topical therapy can reduce burning and stinging; e.g., aerosolized 0.5% bupivacaine or a paste of aluminum hydroxide-magnesium hydroxide.
- Minor bleeding: epistaxis
  1. Avoid disruption of crusted scabs in nose
  2. Keep patient in high-Fowler position with head slightly bent forward
  3. Provide constant pressure to outer nares for 5 to 10 minutes
  4. Apply cold compresses to nape of neck
  5. Provide cool mist humidification to room air to reduce drying of nasal passages
  6. Provide humidification of prescribed nasal oxygen if bleeding occurs from dry nasal passages
  7. NeoSynephrine nasal spray up to qid: DO NOT blow nose after spray
- Minor bleeding: topical sites
  1. Obtain medical orders and instruct caregiver in use of coagulant products, as indicated:
     a. Gelfoam sponge or powder to bleeding site, follow package directions: Moisten Gelfoam sponge with sterile normal saline; apply damp sponge to bleeding wound with moderate pressure until hemostasis results; sponge may be left in place at the site, where it will dissolve, or fresh pieces may be used as needed
     b. Silver nitrate sticks topically to bleeding site if well localized; hold stick to bleeding point followed by a gentle rotation motion
- Moderate to major bleeding

1. Prepare a "hemorrhage kit" with basin, dark towels, blue absorbent chucks, latex gloves, washcloths, trash bags, etc., and keep kit under or near bed for any potential massive hemorrhage
2. Notify physician of frank bleeding episode

NOTE: Where routine topical approaches, such as pressure, epinephrine-soaked gauze, gelfoam, and similar treatments are unsuccessful, not tolerated, or impractical, yet bleeding is continuous and profuse enough to cause distress, pharmacotherapy using fibrinolytic inhibitors may be indicated, per preferences and goals of the patient.

    a. Tranexamic acid: 1.5 g PO loading dose followed by 1 g PO tid
    b. Aminocaproic acid: 5 g PO loading dose followed by 1 g PO qid
3. Apply pressure to bleeding site if appropriate
4. Change saturated dressings as needed
5. Camouflage obvious blood loss if possible
6. Use dark-colored towels to absorb blood
7. Cover urinary drainage bag in presence of gross hematuria
8. Remove soiled dressings or bed clothing as soon as possible
9. Irrigate Foley catheter with normal saline to maintain patency if urinary bleeding
10. Instruct caregiver(s) on universal precautions and handling of bodily fluids (see Section Two   Safety Concerns)
11. Obtain orders for anxiolytic medications (see Section Three—Agitation and Anxiety). Diazepam injectable for IM use may be the most expedient approach if the patient is experiencing significant emotional distress with potentially fatal bleeding

Psychosocial

- Explain what to expect if bleeding does occur and explain purpose of "hemorrhage kit"
- Inform caregiver that bleeding episodes may be accompanied by symptoms of anxiety, restlessness, cool moist skin, and increased pallor
- Instruct caregiver to call hospice nurse or extended coverage staff if hemorrhage should occur
- In the event of brisk bleeding, stay with patient/caregiver
- Initiate continuous care until bleeding is controlled or stops
- Explain option to transfer patient to a contracted facility if the caregiver or patient is extremely anxious and unlikely to cope with impending situation

Goals/Outcomes

- Minimize emotional distress and social isolation
- Reduce or stop bleeding from all sites to the extent possible

- Maintain patient's red cell mass/oxygen carrying capacity in order to prevent anemia-related fatigue and to avoid or minimize the need for palliative red cell transfusion
- Prevent caregiver avoidance of patient
- Facilitate reasoned self-determination about various approaches to therapy for symptomatic blood loss, especially in the consideration of palliative transfusion
- Prevent panic in the event of frank hemorrhage

Documentation in the Medical Record

Initial Medical and Psychosocial Assessment

- Causes and severity of malodorous lesions/sources and bleeding
- Patient/caregiver reaction(s) to malodorous lesions/sources and bleeding
- Likelihood of hemorrhagic event
- Symptoms/signs of anemia

Interdisciplinary Progress Notes

- Content of discussions and results of interventions
- Results of ongoing assessments

IDT Care Plan

- Proposed interventions and contingency plans
- Schedule of reassessments

Confusion/Delirium

SITUATION: Change in mental status with acute confusion that interferes with ability to carry out activities of daily living, patient safety, and adds to caregiver burden

Causes

Biomedical

- Systemic infection (e.g., common occurrence in the elderly with urinary tract infection)
- Dehydration
- Toxic drug reactions (e.g., anticholinergic effects from scopolamine, tricyclic antidepressants, antiemetics, sedatives)
- Organic brain syndrome from underlying disease (e.g., AIDS dementia, neoplasm, cerebrovascular accident)
- Metabolic derangement (e.g., hypercalcemia, hyper/hypoglycemia, electrolyte imbalance, uremia, thyroid dsyfunction, adrenal disease)
- Acute abstinence syndrome (alcohol, opioids, benzodiazapines)

Psychosocial/Spiritual

- Psychological decompensation from stress
- Depression ("pseudo-dementia")
- Fear
- Anxiety
- Pathological grief reaction in anticipation of loss

Findings

Biomedical

- Stigmata of coexisting disease to be found during systemic review and physical examination
- Decreased or increased level of activity, i.e., somnolent versus restless/agitated

Psychosocial

- Alterations in perception and cognition, i.e., decreased or fluctuating level of consciousness, disorientation, and misperception (may only become evident after a long discussion or several visits with the patient)

Evaluation

Biomedical

- Review medications for drugs that may cause or contribute to confusion, especially recently added psychotropic agents or changes in drug or dosing schedule.
- Assess for metabolic derangement based on likelihoods (e.g., blood sugar abnormalities in a known diabetic)
- Associated signs and symptoms
  o Uremia: oliguria/anuria; "frost" on facial skin
  o Hyperglycemia: polydipsia, polyuria, blurred vision, "fruity" odor to breath
  o Hypoglycemia: lethargy to unarousability, tachycardia, diaphoresis
  o Hypercalcemia: polydipsia, polyuria, nausea, ileus, muscle twitching
- Relative burdens (intrusiveness and costs of tests) versus benefits (likelihood of improvement from specific therapeutic interventions)
- Assess for presence of fever or common sources of infection: urinary, respiratory, skin (cellulitis)
- Assess for signs of neurological change to suggest brain metastasis:
  o Volatile mood/behavior or fluctuating level of consciousness, hallucinations, thought disorder
  o Headache
  o Nausea/vomiting
  o Visual impairment (double vision; field cut)
  o Motor, sensory, coordination alteration or deficit
  o Papilledema
- Assess for withdrawal symptoms from alcohol or other drugs:

- o Time of last dose or drink
- o Tachycardia, tachypnea, diaphoresis, hypertension
- o Nausea, abdominal pain, diarrhea
- o Pupillary dilitation (mydriasis)
- o Restlessness, hallucinosis, paranoia

Psychosocial

- Perform Mini-Mental Status Examination (compare with previous baseline if available)
  - o Orientation (person, place, time, situation)
  - o Remote and recent memory (last four presidents, childrens'/grandchildrens' names/birthdates, ability to recall four items after 5 to 10 minutes)
  - o Cognitive function (ability to read simple text and comprehend it; ability to subtract serial 7s from 100; ability to tell time)
  - o Reasoning (what would you do if you smelled smoke in the house?)
  - o Abstraction (what does "people who live in glass houses shouldn't throw stones" mean?)
  - o Spatial integrity (draw a round clock face with numbers and hands)
  - o Assess for presence of insomnia
  - o Assess for presence of delusions and/or hallucinations

Processes of Care

Practical

- Instruct caregiver(s) on reality orientation (frequent reminders of time and place; provide cues such as large-numbered calendar and clock)
- Allay fear: use of night light; familiar objects and persons; patient's favorite music and aromas
- Instruct caregiver(s) on need for simple, structured routine and quiet, calm environment as much as possible

Biomedical

- Provide interventions to ensure adequate periods of rest
- Medicate according to need for patient safety, to relieve distressing symptoms and to obtain reasonable periods of rest, per physician orders
- Notify attending physician if assessment indicates an etiology that is new or imminently treatable
- Pharmacotherapy for palliation of delirium/agitation unrelieved by primary therapies or milieu therapy
  1. Haloperidol 0.5 to 1.0 mg po q6hr; titrate upward as needed
  2. Follow guidelines in Section Three—Agitation and Anxiety if confusional state progresses to a more severe state of agitation

Psychosocial

- Provide a quiet environment: reduce unnecessary noise, activity, clutter
- Speak clearly in simple short sentences; avoid complex explanations; be sure patient can hear you
- Direct patient's attention on the present
- Identify and focus on patient's strengths
- Involve social worker early to assist patient and caregiver with coping skills and to identify need for volunteers and other expertise within the IDT
- Provide support to caregiver
  - o Anticipate cognitive changes with disease progression and educate caregivers to report early, potentially reversible alternations in mental status
  - o Believe caregiver's observations about changes in patient's mental state (these may be subtle to outside observers only seeing patient on an occasional basis)
  - o Arrange for volunteer to relieve family
  - o Assist family to schedule rest periods, so that someone is resting when another is with the patient
  - o Allow caregiver to voice concerns, sadness, and/or anger regarding change in patient's personality

Goals/Outcomes

- Patient is able to rest comfortably without excessive fear, agitation, or restlessness
- Maximize patient's ability to communicate needs and express feelings
- Caregiver burden is minimized to allow adequate periods of rest, sleep, and uninterrupted household activities
- Safe environment is provided for patient and caregiver
- Prevent unnecessary transfers

Documentation in the Medical Record

Initial Medical Assessment

- Precipitating factors leading to confusion
- Signs and symptoms of concurrent or progressive disease
- Findings from systems review and physical examination
- Differential diagnosis of etiology of acute signs/symptoms

Initial Psychosocial Assessment

- Patient behaviors and results of mental status examination
- Goals of therapy and advance directives reviewed/discussed

- Results of interventions
- Observations from repeated assessments
- Caregiver coping

IDT Care Plan

- Order of evaluation and treatment approaches
- Specific interventions
- Contingency plans

Constipation

SITUATION: Decreased bowel motility with consequent constipation, distention, obstipation, or impaction

Causes

- Decreased autonomic function due to aging
- Decreased activity
- Alterations in food and fluid intake
- Inaccessibility of toilet due to decreased mobility, sedation, etc., leading to retention of stool
- Pharmacological effects of opioid analgesics and drugs with anticholinergic activity (e.g., tricyclic antidepressants)
- Painful anorectal lesions (e.g., hemorrhoids, fissures) leading to retention of stool
- Weakness due to primary disease or secondary to asthenia
- Hypokalemia; hypercalcemia

Findings

- Patient report or caregiver assessment of decreased bowel movement frequency, hard stool, or painful elimination
- Soiling of clothing due to seepage of liquid stool around impacted stool in rectum
- Sense of bloating with abdominal distention
- Increase or absence of bowel sounds
- No bowel movement for at least 2 days
- Painful anal lesions

Evaluation

- Bowel assessment should be a regular part of every patient visit.
- Determine date of last bowel movement and stool characteristics.
- Review 24-hour food and fluid intake

- Determine patient's ability to respond to urge to defecate (generate adequate bearing down).
- Determine patient's ability to get to toilet or notify caregiver for help in toileting.
- Auscultate and examine abdomen for quality and intensity (or absence) of bowel sounds, masses, and tenderness.
- Observation, percussion, and palpation of abdomen for distention, tympany, and tenderness
- Assess for and rule out urinary retention commonly associated with fecal impaction.
- Determine if new-onset nausea/vomiting, suspicious for bowel obstruction.
- Anorectal examination for lesions, muscle tone, retained stool, impaction

Processes of Care

Practical and Biomedical

- Notify physician if evidence of bowel obstruction
- Convenience (access to facilities), comfort, and privacy (dignity) should be optimized to promote regular bowel movements and prevent retention.
- All patients taking opioid analgesics should be on some form of anticonstipation regimen
- Increase hydration if consistent with patient wishes and benefits would likely outweigh burdens
- Never use motility agents when there are signs or symptoms of bowel obstruction
- Disimpaction and enemas should precede use of motility agents
- Only recommend or allow use of psyllium (e.g., Metamucil) or bulking foods and fiber (fruits, bran, etc.) in active and well-hydrated patients
- Pharmacotherapy for constipation
  o Rectal suppositories should be placed up against wall of the rectum, not in substance of stool
  o Glycerin suppositories for dry, hard, difficult-to-pass stool
  o Starting anticonstipation regimen
    o Senna preparation (e.g., Senakot tabs 1 to 2 tabs PO q HS, and increase up to 4 tabs tid [may substitute 5 ml of liquid Senakot for each tablet]) as needed; or
    o Bisacodyl 5 mg, 1 or 2 tablets PO at HS or bisacodyl 10 mg suppository PR at HS); double, then triple the dose, adding morning and afternoon doses
  o If no bowel movement within 24 to 48 hours, for hard, desiccated stool, add a stool softener, e.g., docusate sodium 250 mg qd to bid
  o If no bowel movement within 48 hours of initiating therapy, use phosphate (Fleet) enema

- If no bowel movement within 72 hours of initiating therapy, repeat rectal examination; if no evidence of bowel obstruction, no impaction, and no result from oil retention enema (4 oz warmed mineral oil or Fleet Mineral Oil Enema) followed by phosphate enema:
  o Magnesium citrate 8 oz PO or mineral oil 30 to 60 ml PO
  o Lactulose 10 to 30 ml PO qd-bid
- Manual disimpaction
  o Apply local anesthetic preparation (e.g., eutectic mixture of local anesthetic [EMLA cream], lidocaine 2% ointment or 4% gel) liberally to external and internal anal mucosa and administer 4 oz of warm mineral oil into rectal vault 15 to 30 minutes prior to digital dilatation and stool removal
  o If this process causes distress, especially when repeat disempaction is required, premedication with lorazepam 1 to 2 mg and the patient's usual breakthrough dose of analgesic 30 to 60 minutes before manual disimpaction will usually produce favorable conditions

Goals/Outcomes

- Painless, regular bowel movements at least every 3 days
- Absence of induced diarrhea and abdominal cramping from bowel regimen
- Confidence in use of opioid analgesics for pain relief without worry over bowel function

Documentation in the Medical Record

Admission Assessment

- Review of bowel function
- Risks of impending bowel dysfunction due to disease, medications, activity, food/fluid intake
- Patient's and/or family caregiver's ability to manage own bowel care
- Physical examination findings
- Medication review
- Dietary assessment

Interdisciplinary Progress Notes

- History of bowel actions and toileting ability
- Use of bowel protocol
- Therapeutic and adverse effects of bowel protocol
- Findings from repeated physical examination

IDT Care Plan

- Progressive implementation of bowel protocol
- Instructions to patient/caregiver
- Schedule of follow-up evaluations of adherence to bowel protocol and reassessments

Coughing

SITUATION: Frequent cough with resultant pain or discomfort, inability to rest, social disruption, and interruption of sleep

Causes

- Pulmonary infection
- COPD
- Decreased mobility
- Weakness with reduced effectiveness of cough (ineffective clearing of airways)
- Sinus infection
- Respiratory system neoplasm
- Pulmonary edema
- Pleural effusion
- Reactive airways disease (asthma)

Findings

- Loose, productive cough
- Dry, nonproductive cough
- Exasperation, exhaustion, chest pain

Evaluation

Biomedical

- History of new-onset versus recurrent versus chronic cough
- Review history of smoking, asthma, occupational factors.
- Obtain history of triggering and relieving factors.
- Assess cough (frequency, quality, intensity, muscle power).
- Assess sputum characteristics (volume, color, purulence).
- Auscultate lungs for adventitious breath sounds (rhonchi, rales, wheezes), diminished breath sounds, pleural rub.
- Check for periphral edema, jugular venous distention, gallup rhythm.
- Rule out associated paroxysmal nocturnal dyspnea or orthopnea.
- Check for use of accessory muscles of respiration, tachypnea, tachycardia, cyanosis.
- Assess for fever.
- Check for sinus tenderness, nasal discharge.

Psychosocial

- Assess impact of cough on mood, sleep, energy, pain, social interaction.

Processes of Care

Biomedical

- Treat specific etiology of cough if identified (e.g., antibiotics, diuretics, bronchodilators)
- Instruct in proper use of nebulizer, if indicated
- Aggressively treat symptoms in concert with the degree of distress being caused
- Increase humidity in patient's environment—cool mist vaporizer in room
- Elevate head
- Palliative pharmacotherapy
    a. Guaifenensin 5 ml PO q4hr prn or 1 to 2 tablets PO q12hr up to 4 tablets/24 hr
    b. Dextromethorphan-containing cough syrup: use as directed (usually 1 to 2 tsp PO q4hr)
    c. Codeine 15 to 30 mg PO q4hr prn

    NOTE: Adjust dose based on other opioid analgesic use and institute constipation prevention/treatment care plan.

    d. Treat insomnia if nocturnal cough unabated by above therapies (refer to Section Three - Insomnia and Nocturnal Restlessness)
- Instruct in appropriate handling and disposal of sputum (refer to Section Two—Safety Concerns)

Goals/Outcomes

- Ability to clear airways and expectorate sputum and bronchopulmonary secretions
- Reduce coughing paroxysms to the extent possible based on the underlying disease.
- Increase periods of rest and uninterrupted sleep.
- Improve social interaction.
- Maximize hygiene.
- Prevent and treat cough-related pain

Documentation in the Medical Record

Initial Assessment

- Findings of cardiopulmonary systems review and physical examination
- Impact of cough on patient/caregiver

Interdisciplinary Progress Notes

- Results of interventions and ongoing assessments

IDT Care Plan

- Specific interventions and associated goals
- Follow-up and contingency plans

Depression

SITUATION: Depressed mood that interferes with patient care or patient/caregiver ability to cope with the dying process

Causes

Biomedical

- Primary affective disorder
- Unrelieved pain
- Uncontrolled distressing symptoms
- Sleep disorder
- Underlying primary disease-related mood disturbance
- Adverse effect of certain medications (e.g., antihypertensive therapy)

Psychosocial/Spiritual

- Anticipatory grief reaction
- Response to actual loss: function, self-image, future, crisis of faith, etc.
- Boredom, social isolation, sense of uselessness/purposelessness/meaninglessness, lack of goals

Findings

Biomedical

- Sleep disturbance
- Uncontrolled pain or other distressing symptoms (e.g., nausea, chronic cough, etc.)
- Vegetative or agitated behaviors
- Inappropriate medication/substance use or frank misuse of mood altering agents (alcohol, psychotropic drugs, analgesics, sedative-hypnotics)

Psychosocial/Spiritual

- Verbal or facial expression of low mood, sadness
- Flat affect, crying, social withdrawal, isolation
- "Vegetative signs," e.g., hypersomnolence, decreased appetite, psychomotor retardation, anhedonia
- Occasional agitation, volatility, flairs of anger
- Self-deprecation, guilt, hopelessness, self-recrimination

Evaluation

Biomedical

- Determine role of underlying disease or uncontrolled symptoms as cause of depression
- Evaluate effect of medications on signs and symptoms of depression

- Directly ask the question: "Are you depressed?" and rate the response using 0-to-5 scale
- Review of past psychiatric history and response to loss or difficult life events
- Understand patient/caregiver's perception of situation
- Differentiate symptoms as a reaction to circumstances from primary affective disorder, if possible: refer to *DSM-IV*
- Identify patient/caregiver's understanding of, and capacity to address, depression
- Assess severity of depression and likelihood of suicide (refer to Section Two - Suicide: Risk, Prevention, Coping When It Happens)
- Assess impact of depression on care and ability to cope
- Facilitate discussion surrounding faith, values, definitions of hope and meaningfulness to determine potential role of spiritual crisis on depressed mood

Processes of Care

Biomedical

- Consult with physician regarding possible contributory medications and adjustments.
- Discuss indications for antidepressant pharmacotherapy during IDT review.
- Pharmacotherapy for treatment of depression:

NOTE: Supportive counseling and empathic listening by members of the IDT (RN, social worker, chaplain, aide[s], physician, volunteers) should complement pharmacotherapy. Selection of antidepressant medications should be based on symptoms, safety, simplicity of dosing, rapidity of response based on prognosis, safety profile, burden of adverse/side effects, and cost.

1. Depression associated with significant sleep disturbance:
   a. Trazadone 50 mg PO HS, titrated up by 50 mg increments as tolerated q3-5days to 400 mg. Monitor closely for efficacy versus adverse effects, e.g., excessive daytime sedation
   b. Sedating tricyclic antidepressants (e.g., amitriptyline, doxepin) are effective alternatives for sleep disturbance, but anticholinergic effects are more problematic, especially with dose escalation to antidepressant levels. Combined use with an SSRI antidepressant (see Section on Depression, below) is recommended. Monitor for metabolic disturbances and drug-drug interactions that can lead to central serotonin toxicity
   c. Remeron 15 mg PO HS, titrated up by 15-mg increments as tolerated every week up to 45 mg

NOTE: A therapeutic antidepressant effect may take several weeks, but improvements in sleep should occur rapidly, especially at lower doses.

2. Depression without significant sleep disturbance:
   a. Psychostimulants (e.g., methylphenidate 2.5 to 10 mg PO every morning and mid-day) for management of acute depression, especially with very limited life expectancy;
   b. Paroxetine 20 mg PO every morning (10 mg every morning in frail, elderly patients) or
   c. Fluoxetine 20 mg PO every morning, or
   d. Sertraline 50 mg PO every morning, or
   e. Venlafaxine 25 mg PO tid

Psychosocial/Practical/Spiritual

- Initiate discussion and promote expression of thoughts and feelings
- Facilitate discussion of losses
- Identify and reflect distortions in thinking
- Help patient/caregiver understand and accept limits imposed by illness and assuage frustration of trying to control the uncontrollable
- Help patient/caregiver identify what areas in their lives are still under their control
- Help identify attainable goals
- Engage patient/caregiver in life review
- Identify and help facilitate social interactions and recreational/distracting activities that may give meaning to daily life
- Determine if any foods give pleasure, regardless of nutritional value, and make available if possible
- Determine patient need to search for meaning in the dying experience and help him/her to find the language to express this
- Understand patient's values and preferences and facilitate these choices during the dying process to the extent possible
- Help patient/caregiver to identify and use positive coping skills
- Seek out and defer to expert medical/psychiatric treatment if signs/symptoms of depression do not respond to first-line approaches or if risk of suicide is high

Goals/Outcomes

- Reduce "vegetative" signs and symptoms
- Patient/caregiver will be able to openly express feelings of loss
- Patient/caregiver will identify strategies to address depression
- Patient/caregiver will report improved sense of well-being and ability to cope
- The processes of life review and addressing issues raised by the level of debility and realizations imposed by progressive disease and foreseeable death will allow the opportunity for personal growth and finding value in the remaining days of life

Documentation in the Medical Record

Initial Assessment

- Description of mood, sleep, activity, patient short-term goals (if any), patient's identified reasons for low mood
- Patient's self-rating of depression (e.g., 0-to-5 scale: 0 = "Good mood; I do not feel sad or depressed at all" and 5 = "My mood is as low as it could possibly be. I find no meaning in my life.")

Interdisciplinary Team Notes

- Description of interventions and results
- Repeat patient-self reports of depression scores (0-to-5 scale).
- Patient short-term (daily/weekly) attainable goals and results

IDT Care Plan

- Interventions planned
- Means to help patient attain stated goals
- Schedule of IDT visits

Diarrhea and Anorectal Problems

SITUATION: Frequent watery or excessively loose stools with or without ano-rectal irritation, pain, or pruritus

Causes

- Overtreatment of constipation (overuse of laxatives)
- Fecal impaction (overflow incontinence)
- Diet-related
- Drug-related
- Infectious (viral, fungal, bacterial, or other consequence of immunosuppression)
- Intermittent bowel obstruction
- Carcinoid tumor
- Post-gastrectomy "dumping" syndrome
- Pancreatic insufficiency
- Post-radiation or chemotherapy syndrome
- Anorectal tumor

Findings

- Frequent liquid stool (more than three or four bowel movements in 24 hours)
- Abdominal cramping
- Hyperactive bowel sounds

- Anal pain, burning, irritation, itching, tenesmus (feeling of incomplete evacuation)

Evaluation

- Determine usual bowel habits and patterns, duration and extent of change.
- Review current medications and bowel regimen (cathartics, laxatives, stool softeners)
- Review dietary intake and past history of bowel disorders
- Determine relationship between current disease process and propensity for bowel dysfunction
- Systems review for concomitant nausea/vomiting/fever/abdominal pain, blood in stool, number of bowel movements, consistency/color/odor/quality of stool (floating or greasy stool, clay-like, etc.)
- Auscultate bowel sounds and gently palpate abdomen for tenderness and liver enlargement
- Visually examine perineum and anus, and perform digital examination to determine presence of fecal impaction
- General examination to determine if patient is dehydrated: tongue and mucous membranes, skin turgor, orthostatic blood pressure/pulse changes

Processes of Care

Practical and Biomedical

- General:
  a. Notify physician if new or rapidly advancing signs/symptoms, e.g., abdominal distention suspected bowel obstruction, gastrointestinal bleeding, severe dehydration, etc
  b. Discontinue cathartics/laxatives until symptoms abate and then reinstitute gradually
  c. Clear fluids with slowly advancing diet as symptoms allow and appetite dictates
  d. Rehydrate orally if possible; otherwise, consider subcutaneous infusion (hypodermoclysis) of normal saline if prognosis warrants, unless absolutely necessary medications cannot be delivered by this route and intravenous access is necessary
- Normal saline with 500 units/L hyaluronidase (only if readily available, to enhance absorption); infuse at 0.5 to 1.0 ml/kg/hr with a maximum rate of 60 ml/hr, using a 25-gauge butterfly needle inserted at a 45-degree angle to the skin, or a subcutaneous "button" device.
  e. Nonspecific pharmacotherapy:
     o Kaopectate 60 ml q2hr until diarrhea stops, or;
     o Loperamide HCl (Imodium AD) 2 to 4 mg PO after each loose stool (1 tablet = 2 mg or 5 ml liquid formulation = 1 mg). If ineffective, try
     o Diphenoxylate HCl (Lomotil) 1 or 2 tablets after each loose stool

- Etiology-specific approaches to therapy:
  a. Carcinoid tumors
     o Octreotide 150 to 300 µg SQ bid or q24hr by continuous infusion
  b. Dumping syndrome (postgastrectomy)
     o Small nonfatty meals
     o Octreotide 150–300 µg SQ bid or up to 750 µg q24hr by continuous infusion
  c. Fungal or other infection or immunosuppression
     o Clotrimazole 10 to 20 mg PO tid or fluconazole 150 mg PO every morning
     o Loperamide 2 to 4 mg PO up to 16 mg/day
     o Diphenoxylate 1 tab PO after each diarrheal stool up to 8 tabs/day
     o Tincture of opium (if available); otherwise, codeine elixir or oral morphine solution titrated to effect
  d. Pancreatic insufficiency
     o Pancreatic enzyme replacement (with meals)
     o Famotidine 20 mg PO bid
     o Loperamide 2 to 4 mg PO up to 16 mg/day
  e. Post radiation or chemotherapy syndrome
     o Eliminate fiber and milk products.
     o NSAIDs (e.g., ibuprofen) for radiation enteritis (see Section Three - Pain) if tolerated
     o Progressive trial of loperamide, diphenoxylate, tincture of opium (if available); otherwise, codeine elixir or oral morphine solution, titrated to control symptoms
     o Octreotide 100 µg SQ bid for otherwise uncontrolled chemotherapy-induced enteritis
  f. Anal irritation
     o Clear warm water nonabrasive cleansing and thorough drying
     o Apply zinc oxide to unbroken skin
     o Apply corticosteroid cream to macerated or inflamed skin 1 to 2 days only
  g. Rectal tumors
     o If prognosis warrants, consider palliative radiation therapy or endoscopic laser therapy.
     o Hydrocortisone foam, 1 applicator PR bid
     o EMLA cream or other topical local anesthetic formulation prn
     o For severe pruritus ani, use a sedating antihistamine, e.g., promethazine 12.5 mg PO HS.

Goals/Outcomes

- Regular well-formed stools to the extent possible, limited only by underlying disease and patient tolerance/preference of interventions.

- Ability to ingest foods of choice without undue discomfort or diarrhea
- Absence of perineal/anal discomfort

Documentation in the Medical Record

Initial Assessment

- Number and character of bowel movements
- Likely etiology of diarrhea
- Contributing factors to diarrhea
- Patient/caregiver approaches to controlling diarrhea
- Findings from physical examination

Interdisciplinary Progress Notes

- Therapies applied and results of interventions
- Findings from reassessment: frequency/quality of bowel movements and associated symptoms; physical examination

IDT Care Plan

- Interventions planned and schedule of re-assessments
- Contingency plans

Dysphagia and Oropharyngeal Problems

SITUATION: Difficult or painful swallowing, mucositis, oral candidiasis (thrush), and other painful or distressing/disturbing oropharyngeal conditions associated with advanced disease

Causes

- Dysphagia, with or without oral candidiasis or mucositis, commonly occurs in patients:
    a. With cancers of the head and neck, gastrointestinal tract, and those involving mediastinal structures
    b. Patients who have undergone radiation treatments to these areas
    c. Patients who are severely immunocompromised (e.g., AIDS, post-chemotherapy, steroid therapy)
    d. Patients who have progressive neuromuscular diseases (e.g., ALS)
    e. Patients who have cerebrovascular disease (post-stroke)
    f. Patients who are experiencing medication-induced dystonic reactions

Findings

- Excessive secretions, drooling
- Painful and/or uncoordinated swallowing
- Avoidance of food or beverages

- Choking
- Panting or other postures indicating difficulty in managing oral secretions and swallowing
- Whitish patches (plaques) in oral cavity (tongue, mucosal surface, gingiva) that scrape off and have a beefy red base
- Erythematous oral mucosa without plaques (atrophic candidiasis)
- Taste perversion

Evaluation

- History and systems review pertinent to upper gastrointestinal system, including sense of taste, quality and intensity of pain, difficulties with chewing and swallowing
- Examination of oropharynx: observe for signs of candida, other lesions, fit of dentures, odor (halitosis)
- Observe patient manage own secretions during history-taking, and observe patient during the act of swallowing
- Review medications for possible dystonic reactions from phenothiazines, butyrophenones, etc. (e.g., prochlorperazine, chlorpromazine, haloperidol, droperidol)

Processes of Care

Practical

- Optimize positioning for drinking and eating (sitting if possible, or elevated head of bed).
- Frequent small sips or meals; crushed ice; refresh bedside beverages/ice frequently
- Cool compress to throat
- Have patient avoid excessively sour (acidic) or hot fluids/meals until symptoms remit. Soft, cool meals (yogurt, cottage cheese, Jello, ice cream) may be all that is tolerated.
- Dietary/nutritionist consultation

Biomedical

- For dystonia, if symptom-causing medication is still indicated, initiate therapy with diphenhydramine 25 to 50 mg PO/IV qid or benztropine 1 to 2 mg PO/IV qd or bid
- For painful oral candidiasis and mucositis, use opioid analgesics as needed to control pain until antifungal therapy has been effective. A 1:2:8 mixture of diphenhydramine elixir:lidocaine (2-4%):Maalox as a swish-and-swallow suspension provides temporary relief of symptoms and might lessen the need for opioid analgesics, especially prior to meal times
- Edema, inflammation, tumor burden: consider corticosteroids and H_2 blockers (potential benefit of corticosteroids must be balanced against associated risks of immunosuppression)

- For candidiasis, treat with:
  1. Topical treatment with clotrimazole 10-mg troches, 5 doses/day can be initiated, as symptoms and patient compliance allow
  2. If symptoms do not rapidly abate, or patient compliance does not allow topical antifungal therapy, fluconazole 150 mg PO followed by 100 mg PO daily for 5 days
- Intractable oral bleeding: if available, apply topical thrombin to hemorrhagic areas. Consider tranexamic acid 500 to 1000 mg PO tid or aminocaproic acid 5 g PO followed by 1 g PO qid (see Section Three - Bleeding, Oozing and Malodorous Lesions)
- Severe halitosis should be treated to prevent reluctance to care, social isolation, humiliation, and nausea.
  1. Frequent prophylactic care (cleansing of dentures and oropharynx)
  2. Antimicrobial mouthwash or half-strength hydrogen peroxide gargle.
  3. Metronidazole 250–500 mg PO tid or applied as a topical gel (0.75%), if feasible, to putrid necrotic or fungating lesions for control of anaerobic colonization (see Section Three - Bleeding, Oozing and Malodorous Lesions)
  4. Broad-spectrum antibiotics (e.g., trimethoprim-sulfa; cephalosporin) for foul-smelling, purulent bronchopulmonary sputum/secretions

Goals/Outcomes

- Decrease pain
- Normalize swallowing and control of secretions as much as disease status allows
- Improve enjoyment of food and beverages
- Improve ability to talk
- Reduce social isolation, embarrassment, nausea

Documentation in the Medical Record

Initial Assessment

- History of difficulty with swallowing or managing secretions, choking
- Type and quantity of food/beverage intake
- Pain in mouth, throat, or mediastinum
- Physical examination findings
- Patient/caregiver ability to cope with symptoms/interventions
- Patient ability to ingest oral or buccal medications; possible need for liquid forms of pills/capsules and/or transdermal, subcutaneous, or intravenous dosage forms

Interdisciplinary Progress Notes

- Interventions recommended and tried
- Results of interventions

- Patient/caregiver difficulties with compliance
- Findings from repeat physical examinations

IDT Care Plan
- Specific interventions for each identified symptom
- Oral hygiene plan
- Contingency plans
- Schedule of follow-up visits/examinations

Edema: Peripheral Edema, Ascites, and Lymphedema

SITUATION: Peripheral edema, ascites, or lymphedema that results in physical or emotional distress, functional impairment, or adds difficulty to caregiving

Causes

- Ascites and lymphedema
  - o Primary neoplasm (ovary, breast, endometrium, colon, stomach, pancreas, bronchus, hepatobiliary)
  - o Metastatis to peritoneum or liver
  - o Venous or lymphatic obstruction/occlusion due to neoplasm
  - o Portal hypertension secondary to advanced liver disease
  - o Chylous ascites (lymph plus emulsified fat and white blood cells) from lymphatic obstruction or abdominal lymphoma
  - o Postsurgical or radiotherapy-induced lymphatic obstruction
- Peripheral edema
  - o Hypoalbuminemia
  - o Chronic steroid therapy
  - o Renal failure
  - o Congestive heart failure
  - o Circulatory impairment from inadequate mobility/prolonged dependency
  - o Fluid overload from artificial nutrition
  - o Chronic peripheral vascular disease/postthrombosis syndrome
  - o Cor pulmonale (right heart failure) due to advanced pulmonary disease
  - o Acute phlebitis

Findings

- Ascites
  - o Feelings of bloating, regurgitation, or reflux
  - o Early satiety and nausea

- o Increased abdominal girth, shifting dullness, fluid wave, "Caput Medusa" (engorged venous plexus visible on abdominal wall in severe cases of portal hypertension)
- o Lower extremity/genital swelling
- o Orthopnea and dyspnea as ascites progresses
- Lymphedema or peripheral edema
  - o Swelling of distal extremities with pitting of skin when gentle pressure is applied
  - o Presence of fluid accumulation in dependent body parts (e.g., presacral area in bed-bound patients)
  - o Unilateral extremity swelling in postsurgical or postradiotherapy lymphedema
  - o Tight and shiny skin with visible fluid extrusion in severe cases
  - o Jugular venous distention
  - o Pain with acute phlebitis
  - o Electrolyte abnormalities

Evaluation

- Assess cardiovascular status, e.g., vital signs, cardiac rate, rhythm, murmurs, rubs, gallups, jugular veins, peripheral pulses, peripheral perfusion
- Examine dependent body parts and extremities
- Auscultate lungs for rales, rubs, and decreased breath sounds
- Examine abdomen for findings of ascites
- Assess fluid balance (volume in, urine out); when appropriate; consider benefit-burden of serum electrolyte and protein assessment
- Assess weight changes, when feasible
- Assess for tachypnea and respiratory distress
- Evaluate for symptoms of reflux
- Determine association between body position and physical signs and symptoms of distress

Processes of Care

Practical and Biomedical

- Ascites: Pharmacotherapy to reduce the ascitic burden should be tried, but effects may be marginal, especially in malignant ascites.
  1. Diuretics
     a. Spironolactone 100 mg PO daily up to 200 mg bid. If needed, add
     b. Furosemide 40 to 240 mg PO daily. Continuous infusion of 100 mg/24 hr IV is an alternative. Balance benefits against potential adverse effects, such as volume depletion and electrolyte disturbance.
  2. Very tense or clinically distressing ascites that is intractable to diuretic therapy may require bedside paracentesis by the physician to relieve excessively

burdensome symptoms that are poorly controlled by less invasive means. If highly symptomatic ascites reaccumulates quickly, and the patient is not imminently dying, discussion regarding the placement of a dialysis catheter for continuous drainage, acknowledging the burdens associated with such a procedure (transport to a day-surgery facility; discomfort from the operative procedure; risk of infection, occlusion, dislodgment).

- Lymphedema: primary treatment consists of nonpharmacological approaches (e.g., postural support; maintaining range of motion with active or passive physical therapy, as tolerated; compression bandaging/gloves/stockings/pneumatic devices). Diuretics (per Section Three—Dyspnea, above) should be tried if symptoms are distressing, although responses to drug therapy are not generally very positive
- Peripheral edema
  - o Review current diuretic and cardiac medications with physician, and adjust appropriately (see above)
  - o Elevate legs prn unless contraindicated by compromised cardiac function.
  - o Turn and reposition recumbent patients q2hr as tolerated.
  - o Consider relative benefits/burdens of decreasing fluid intake.
  - o Consider need for daily potassium supplement when patient is on long-term diuretic therapy
  - o Consider antibiotic therapy if cellulitis is present.
  - o Notify physician if findings of acute thrombophlebitis are present.

Goals/Outcomes

- Reduce ascites, lymphedema, and peripheral edema to the greatest extent with the least invasive approaches possible in order to minimize physical and emotional distress, improve patient physical functioning, and facilitate caregiving.

Documentation in the Medical Record

Initial Assessment

- Results of systems review and physical examination
- Intensity and types of physical and emotional distress, functional loss to patient imposed by ascites/lymphedema/peripheral edema
- Degree of burden imposed by untreated signs/symptoms on caregiver

Interdisciplinary Progress Notes

- Content of discussion regarding treatment options
- Types and results of interventions

IDT Care Plan

- Defined goals of therapies
- Specific interventions and contingency plans

Fatigue, Weakness (Aesthenia), and Excessive Sedation

SITUATION: The patient's quality of life is severely impacted by fatigue, weakness, or diminished energy due to advancing disease.

Causes

- Most chronic disease states in the far advanced stages (e.g., cancer, COPD, heart failure, renal failure, hepatic failure) lead to a state of aesthenia, characterized by chronic fatigue and weakness. These continue to be some of the most challenging symptoms to manage effectively, once pain is under control.
- Catabolic nutritional state due to disease factors
- Hypoxemia or inadequate oxygen-carrying capacity (decreased red cell mass)
- Clinical depression should be ruled out since the symptoms of depression may mimic aesthenia (see Section Three - Depression)
- Boredom: absence of stimulation is very common in homebound and especially bedridden patients, and can mimic depression

Findings

- Weakness, lethargy, fatigue, hypersomnolence after minimal or no activity

Evaluation

Biomedical

- Simple measures to find reversible or easily treatable causes of severe fatigue, lethargy, and weakness (e.g., metabolic disturbances, anemia, hypoxemia) should be sought and treated when the context is appropriate (i.e., life expectancy will allow meaningful benefit from testing and therapeutic intervention). In patients with rapid decline from life-limiting diseases, the luxury of an exhaustive evaluation is not always feasible or in the patient's best interest. In these cases, or where reversible processes are not present or specifically directed therapies are not possible, empiric therapy is indicated.
- Review current medications and determine if there are any changes which, on balance, might lead to overall benefits
- Evaluate muscle tone and strength. Unless myopathic weakness is the result of ongoing corticosteroid therapy, this class of drugs can palliate symptoms of weakness and fatigue for a short duration of time (days to weeks)

Psychosocial/Spiritual

- Determine patient/caregiver perceptions and level of distress imposed by degree of fatigue and weakness

- Determine to what degree important short-term goals are being impeded by symptoms

Processes of Care

Biomedical

- Consider and discuss benefits and burdens of red cell transfusion if anemia is a likely contributing cause of symptoms
- Use supplemental oxygen only if a therapeutic trial proves beneficial when hypoxemia is determined to be the cause of symptoms
- In patients with heart failure, review medical management and determine if there are any adjustments in cardiotropic drugs that may improve end-organ perfusion, balancing benefits/burdens and patient preferences
- Palliative pharmacotherapy using psychostimulants can be tried. The use of dextroamphetamine or methylphenidate may be especially useful in balancing therapeutic analgesic effects of opioids against excessive daytime sedation. Modafinil has also been reported to be beneficial, although cost is appreciably higher than that of other psychostimulants; it should be considered if other modalities are not well tolerated. Close follow-up and monitoring for incipient signs of psychosis, agitation, or sleep disturbance are obligatory when instituting these drug therapies:

1. Dextroamphetamine* 2.5 mg PO every morning to start or;
2. Methylphenidate* 2.5 PO every morning to start or;
3. Modafinil 200 mg PO every morning

Psychosocial/Spiritual

- Provide realistic information about the natural history of the disease process being experienced, with aesthenia being a usual and expected consequence
- Help organize the patient/caregiver routines to conserve energy and pace activities
- Help set limits on social visits if they seem to be more exhausting than helpful.
- Help reset goals to a level that is more attainable based on the patient's capabilities
- Consider occupational therapy evaluation to determine if there is any form of stimulation that might be beneficial; utilize volunteers to carry on such a program to intercede against boredom

Goals/Outcomes

- Maximize patient energy based on the course of disease, in keeping with patient preferences

---

*These medications can be upward titrated as needed and can be used as often as 3 to 4 times per day, depending on each patient's needs and response to therapy. There is some evidence that small doses throughout the day may be more effective than morning and mid-day dosing and do not lead to insomnia as has been traditionally thought.

- Decreased frustration with clinical circumstances beyond patient/caregiver/professional control
- Patient feels free from having to perform at an unrealistic level of expectation
- Identify short-term goals (whatever they are—even simply "being") that are attainable and lead the patient to feel that his/her existence has value

Documentation in the Medical Record

Initial Assessment

- Description of patient's level of fatigue, functional capabilities
- Determination if goals and expectations are realistic
- Degree of acceptance versus frustration with clinical circumstances
- Identification of factors contributing to fatigue, weakness (pacing, length of social visits, structure and schedule of activities throughout the day)

Interdisciplinary Progress Notes

- Content of discussions, ongoing evaluations, interventions
- Results of interventions

IDT Care Plan

- Specific interventions and role of IDT members in helping to manage coping issues

Fever and Diaphoresis

SITUATION: Fever and/or diaphoresis associated with terminal illness

Causes

- Infection
- Tumor-related pyrexia
- Tumor-related nocturnal afebrile diaphoresis (night sweats)
  o Lymphoma
  o Certain lung cancers
- Drug-induced afebrile diaphoresis (e.g., morphine)
- Central nervous system metastasis or primary neoplasm
- Drug- or transfusion-related pyrogenic reaction
- Dehydration

Findings

- Elevated body temperature (above 100.5° F orally, 99.5° F axillary, 101.5° F rectally)
- Flushed warm skin, generalized aching, irritability
- Tachycardia

- Altered mental status (decreased level of consciousness or agitation/restlessness, fitful sleep)
- Diaphoresis (sweating) with or without fever

Evaluation

- Systems review and physical examination to rule out infection (e.g., urinary tract, respiratory tract, cellulitis)
- Stage and extent of disease in relation to cause of fever/diaphoresis
- Recent medication change as potential cause of fever/diaphoresis

Processes of Care

Practical

- Increase room air circulation and give cool sponge baths
- Cool wet towels or ice packs to groin and axilla for temperature above 103°F as symptoms dictate and if tolerated
- Remove heavy bed clothes and bedding
- Provide mouth care: use toothette dipped in fluid of choice to moisten mouth and apply lip balm to keep lips from cracking

Biomedical

- Empiric broad-spectrum antibiotic therapy ONLY if occult or obvious infection is suspected AND symptoms are a cause of significant discomfort or a major burden to caregivers (e.g., necessity for frequent bedclothes changes).
- Pharmacotherapeutic approaches
  1. Antipyretics
     a. Acetaminophen 5 to 10 mg/kg PO/PR q4-6hr around the clock, or;
     b. NSAIDs (e.g., ibuprofen 10 mg/kg PO q8hr or naproxyn sodium 4 mg/kg PO q8hr)
  2. Treatment of rigors (shaking chills) is empiric. Some recommended approaches are:
     a. Meperidine 0.25 to 0.5 mg/kg IV/IM/SQ prn (*NOTE: this is an exception to the usual injunction against the use of meperidine*), or;
     b. Promethazine 12.5 to 25 mg PO/IM/IV or 25 to 50 mg PR q6-8hr prn
  3. For suspected metastasis-induced diaphoresis (e.g., liver metastasis) or morphine-induced sweating:
     a. Dexamethasone 2 mg PO, or;
     b. Indomethacin 50 mg PR q12hr
  4. For prevention of macerated skin:
     a. Zinc oxide paste applied to intertriginous areas and other at-risk sites

Goals/Outcomes

- Reduce fever- and diaphoresis-associated discomfort and distress
- Decrease sleep disruption
- Minimize caregiving burden

Documentation in the Medical Record

Initial Assessment

- Body temperature and associated signs and symptoms of fever
- Timing of fever, diaphoresis (day/night)
- Interventions (and results) attempted by caregiver
- Differential diagnosis based on history and physical examination

Interdisciplinary Progress Notes

- Effect of interventions on symptoms

IDT Care Plan

- Specific interventions and contingency plans

Hiccups

SITUATION: Pain or discomfort and exhaustion due to persistent hiccups

Causes

- Gastric dysmotility with distention due to extrinsic obstruction or intrinsic disease
- Phrenic or vagus nerve irritation due to tumor or inflammation
- Cerebral neoplasms, metastasis or other central nervous system disorders, e.g., cerebrovascular disesase
- Metabolic disturbances, e.g., uremia, hypocalcemia, hyponatremia
- Sepsis
- Manifestation of anxiety disorder

Findings

- Disruption of social interactions, eating, sleep
- Reflux esophagitis ("heartburn")
- Occasional cause of aspiration due to reflux
- Anxiety, aerophagia

Evaluation

Biomedical

- Systems review and physical examination for disease-related etiology as described earlier
- Metabolic evaluation in patients with an extended life expectancy where specific interventions to remediate the disorder are feasible should be discussed with the physician, IDT, and patient
- Effect of hiccups on pain, sleep

- Association of hiccups to secondary disorders such as reflux and aspiration
- Determine relationship of hiccups episodes to position, medication use, and type of food intake.

Psychosocial

- Assess anxiety and "air swallowing" (aerophagia) as well as relationship of hiccups to sleep; hiccups that occur ONLY during wakefulness point to psychological causes.

Process of Care Delivery

Practical

- Nonpharmacological management techniques often suffice, but they may require repetition. These include various means of trying to stimulate nasopharyngeal reflexes and associated cranial nerves involved in the hiccup reflex arc, e.g.:
  o Swallowing or applying granulated sugar under the tongue
  o Insertion of a small flexible catheter gently through the nose into the posterior pharynx
  o Elevating the uvula with a cotton-tipped applicator
  o Drinking from the far side of a glass (difficult for very ill patients to understand or carry out)
  o Cold application to the back of the neck
  o Breathing into paper bag
- Elevate the head of the bed, or support patient in a semirecumbent position with pillows/bolsters, especially after meals
- Experiment with position changes to determine if any one position offers relief, e.g,, lateral.

Biomedical

- Adjunctive use of pharmacotherapy to maintain a "remission" from recurrent bouts of hiccups might be necessary. All of the following drug regimens have been found to be effective, but each patient requires a trial-and-error approach. Start with the least toxic and least likely side effect-inducing course of therapy (this also depends on each patient's unique set of circumstances) and substitute for the next treatment on the list if needed.

  1. Metoclopramide 10 to 20 mg PO/IV qid if there is delayed gastric emptying ***without bowel obstruction***
  2. Simethicone and/or charcoal-containing antacids prn
  3. Haloperidol 1 to 5 mg PO/IV qid, or chlorpromazine 10 to 25 mg PO or 25 mg suppository PR qid
  4. Prednisone 1 mg/kg/day, then taper, if hepatomegaly or tumor effect is suspected as etiology
  5. Diazapam 2 to 10 mg PO qid prn
  6. Baclofen 5 to 15 mg PO q6-8hr prn
  7. Phenytoin 100 mg PO bid

Psychosocial
- Treat anxiety as described in "Agitation and Anxiety."

Goals/Outcomes
- Reduce or eliminate episodes of hiccuping to the extent possible without incurring additional symptom burdens from treatment
- Provide periods of uninterrupted rest and sleep
- Improve social interaction and ability to partake of meals as per patient preference
- Eliminate "heartburn" and risk of aspiration

Documentation in the Medical Record
Initial Assessment
- Frequency and duration of hiccup episodes with inciting and relieving factors, if identified
- Putative etiology of hiccups, if identified
- Effect of hiccups on social interaction, meals, pain, sleep, mood

Interdisciplinary Progress Notes
- Effects of interventions

IDT Care Plan
- Decisions regarding value of further medical work-up
- Specific interventions (nonmedical and medical) with contingency and follow-up plans

Imminent Death

SITUATION: Rapid decline in medical condition with associated signs and symptoms of imminent death

Findings
- Overall deterioration of bodily functions/homeostasis with accompanying general systems failure
- Cardiac, hepatic, renal, pulmonary failure with associated fluid and electrolyte disturbances
- Deterioration of cognition and higher brain functions
- Progressive circulatory failure
- In some cases, there may be a distinct but prolonged phase of systems failure lasting a week or more, characterized by:
  - Diminished appetite
  - Decreased urinary output
  - Progressive lethargy (obtundation)

Section Three: Clinical Processes and Symptom Management

- o   Social withdrawal
- o   Speaking to being(s) unseen by others in attendance
- o   Picking at bed clothes or in the air
- o   Agitation or restlessness
- In other cases, when death is not a sudden event, the phase of imminent dying is shorter, lasting 2 to 3 days, and this period of time is often characterized by:
  - o   Tachypnea with periods of apnea (Cheyne-Stokes respirations)
  - o   Increased use of accessory muscles for respiration
  - o   Tachycardia
  - o   Hypotension
  - o   Weak peripheral pulses
  - o   Cool, mottled extremities
  - o   Terminal congestion ("death rattle")
  - o   Terminal restlessness or agitation

Evaluation

- Assess the need for support by various members of the IDT, depending on areas of expertise, especially the need for spiritual and bereavement support
- Anticipate the mode of death in order to prepare family/caregiver
- Assess for behaviors suggestive of pain, dyspnea, fear
- Determine whether bladder emptying is taking place
- Determine type of secretions causing "death rattle"
  - o   Oral: clear, relatively thin, not particularly malodorous
  - o   Bronchial: purulent, relatively thick, fetid odor
- Assess caregiver's level of comfort, capability and competency with basic cares, e.g., hygiene, positioning, suctioning, medication administration
- Determine if postdeath plans have been made (funeral home, etc.)
- Review with caregiver if important family members/significant others need to be or want to be notified of patient status
- Determine whether current level of care is sufficient to manage patient symptoms and/or support caregiver

Processes of Care

Practicaland Biomedical

- Review and ensure provision of basic processes of physical care: oropharyngeal care (lips, teeth, oral mucosa), bathing, positioning, skin care, suctioning, medication administration
- Ensure adequacy of urinary drainage, if urine is still being produced
- Nonpurulent secretions: a patient's inability to control or swallow secretions can be managed by positioning and having suction available for use by the caregivers coupled with the use of drying agents when respiratory

sounds are disturbing to those close to the patient. There are many choices for palliative pharmacotherapy. Convenience, cost, potential for undesirable (adverse or toxic) effects should lead to the most rational first choice, with appropriate monitoring and adjustments made based on response.

1. Transdermal scopolamine patches: each patch delivers 1 mg of scopolamine per 24 hours for 3 days. More than one patch may be required, titrating therapeutic effects against potential side effects, which include sedation and delirium.
2. Hyoscyamine 0.125 mg SL q1-2hr prn
3. Scopolamine 0.3 to 0.6 mg SQ prn
4. Glycopyrrolate 0.2 mg IV/SQ prn
5. Atropine 1 to 2 mg IM/SQ/SL/nebulized q4hr or prn

- Purulent secretions should also be managed with positioning and suctioning, but drying agents may not be particularly helpful. A single IM/IV injection of a broad spectrum antibiotic (e.g., a cephalosporin such as cefotaxime 500 to 1000 mg IM/IV) has been shown to sufficiently decrease the bacterial count with accompanying elimination of malodorous character of bronchial secretions. This effect may last for days, allowing a much reduced caregiving burden and eliminate a barrier to physical closeness
- Restlessness or agitation: refer to "Agitation and Anxiety."
- Change route of medication administration if oral route has been in effect and this route is no longer feasible: consult with physician/pharmacist as necessary for dosage conversions/formulations if not already prearranged
- Notify primary care (referring) physician and/or hospice physician of status, depending on expressed preferences
- Institute appropriate level of care to ensure adequate symptom management and essential cares

Psychosocial/Spiritual/Practical

- Continue to reassure patient through verbal communication and touch, even if no direct evidence of understanding or acknowledgment by the patient
- Offer emotional support to caregiver, answer questions, and provide situation-specific information about processes of dying including:
  o Possible occurrence of death during turning or other basic cares
  o Possible occurrence of death during transport to another care facility if that becomes the choice/preference/necessity
  o Possible occurrence of a post-mortem audible exhalation
- Help to distinguish and give reassurance to the caregiver and others in attendance about the difference between pain/suffering and terminal vocalizations, if present

- Reassure caregiver/family that discontinuation of food/fluids when patient is no longer interested or responsive is "best care," reducing the burden to patient
- Institute appropriate level of care to ensure adequate patient and caregiver support
- Help to notify designated family, friends, clergy, etc., per patient/caregiver preferences
- Review contingency plans for caregiver coping/support, e.g., 24-hour hospice telephone number in order to prevent a "panic" reaction such as dialing 911
- Review information on procedure to follow after death, including disposition of body to funeral home or other prearrangements
- Provide mouth and eye care: use toothette dipped in fluid of choice to moisten mouth and apply lip balm to keep lips from cracking; use artificial tears to moisten eyes, if open, and warm water and soft cloth to clear mucous/crusting
- Facilitate and respect rituals as specified by patient/family

Goals/Outcomes

The dying process and death itself will occur with maximal comfort and with dignity. Caregiver/family will experience a sense of enduring emotional comfort from the experience of their loved one dying in a nurturing/caring environment and in a manner that respected their preferences to the greatest extent possible

Documentation in the Medical Record

Initial Assessment

- Determination that on initial assessment the patient is imminently dying
- Focus of the evaluation should be on biomedical/psychosocial/practical/spiritual findings and preparation for death.

Interdisciplinary Progress Notes

- Ongoing and progressive physical signs and symptoms
- Coping by caregiver/family
- Description of instructions, preparations, interventions
- Results of interventions

IDT Care Plan

- Specific interventions planned
- Contingency plans and schedule of follow-up by various members of IDT
- Updated bereavement plan

Insomnia and Nocturnal Restlessness

SITUATION: Disturbed sleep or significant alteration in sleep pattern interfering with patient sense of well-being or adding to caregiver burden

Causes

Difficulty falling asleep, frequent awakening, early morning awakening, and non-refreshing sleep are prevalent symptoms in the general population, and become even more frequent and burdensome with chronic, progressive diseases. Poor sleep impacts greatly on mood, coping abilities, pain tolerance, interpersonal relations, appetite, energy, and overall sense of well-being. Some of the usual contributors to sleep disturbance that are important to identify in order to tailor therapy appropriately and specifically are:

- Poorly controlled pain or other physical symptoms such as "heartburn," nausea, pruritus, dyspnea, diarrhea, urinary frequency
- Hypoxemia
- Depression (can be a cause and a result of sleep disturbance)
- Anxiety, worries, fretfulness, fears
- Unresolved intrapersonal, spiritual or relationship issues/conflicts
- Nocturnal delirium and disorientation ("sun-downing")
- "Activating" medications or paradoxical effects from medications
- Ingestion of stimulants, such as caffeine or other methylxanthine-containing beverages/foods
- Use of tobacco products
- Reversal of sleep-wakefulness cycles by inactivity and napping during the day

Findings

- Complaint of poor sleep, exhaustion
- Cognitively functional and expressive patients may be able to report on sleep history but many patients are not aware of the details of sleep disturbance or nocturnal behaviors, requiring reliance on caregiver reports and/or daytime symptoms.
- Moodiness, grouchiness, emotional lability/volatility
- Daytime sedation, night-time restlessness
- Caregiver fatigue, exasperation, "burnout"

Evaluation

Biomedical

- Obtain sleep history
  - Sleep-preceding activities, food/fluid intake, toileting, medications, relaxation techniques, etc.
  - Time until sleep is initiated

- o Times and frequency, duration of wakeful periods
- o Nocturnal behaviors/signs/symptoms (e.g., pain/discomfort, agitation, rest-lessness, out of bed, toileting, air hunger, panic, anxiety, nightmares/terrors, diaphoresis, thirst/hunger)
- Assess for dementia
- Assess for adequacy of medical management for congestive heart failure and COPD
- Assess for past history of restless legs syndrome or other sleep-related movement disorders (periodic leg movements)

Psychosocial/Spiritual

- Assess for anxiety, depression, panic disorder
- Evaluate contributors such as fear (for self or others), intra/interpersonal conflicts (e.g., unresolved anger, guilt), spiritual concerns
- Assess caregiver level of fatigue and coping strategies

Practical

- Assess sleeping quarters/environment/bed/pillows/bedclothes, etc
- Assess safety concerns (see Section Two - Living Environment, Finances and Support Systems)
- Assess caregiver support at night and ability to rest during the day
- Determine if level of care is sufficient to provide adequate care throughout the day and night

Processes of Care
Practical

- Progressive relaxation techniques/exercises to the extent possible
- Small carbohydrate bedtime snack/beverage; warm milk with favorite flavoring

  NOTE: An alcoholic beverage may be useful for some patients but be aware of possible rebound effects (reawakening within 1 to 2 hours), increased reflux/heartburn symptoms, and diuretic effects.

- Presleep talk, story-telling, music per patient preference
- Ensure a safe environment
- Maximize daytime activities and limit daytime napping to the extent possible
- Increase level of care to provide intense symptom management and/or respite as indicated

Biomedical

- Optimize medical management of dyspnea, PND, orthopnea; elevate head of bed
- Treat hypoxemia (trial of oxygen therapy; only continue if clearly beneficial)

- Treat anemia (if profound and symptomatic, and expected duration of life warrants transfusion or pharmacotherapy)
- Treat symptoms of reflux (see Section Three - Dysphagia and Oropharyngeal Problems)
- Treat continuous and breakthrough pain (see Section Three - Pain)
- Eliminate pharmacological/dietary contributors
- Treat restless legs syndrome (if not caused by hypoxemia/anemia/ischemia).
  o Low-dose sedating tricyclic antidepressant medication (e.g., amitriptyline, doxepin), starting at 10 mg PO HS, titrated slowly to effect; monitor for anticholinergic adverse effects
  o Low-dose Sinemet (10 to 100) [review pharmacology and contraindications before initiating therapy]
  o Gabapentin, starting at 100 mg PO HS, with upward titration as tolerated to determine effectiveness at reducing sleep-disturbing symptoms without inducing daytime side effects
  o Ropinirole (starting at 0.25 mg HS, with upward dose titration every 3 to 5 days as needed, up to 4 mg) is the only drug specifically approved for this condition, but less costly approaches may be warranted first
- Treat severe anxiety, depression, panic disorder, agitation if not adequately responsive to nonpharmacological interventions
- Initiate pharmacotherapy for insomnia as required, based on response to nonpharmacological interventions:

NOTE: There is a risk of increasing confusion, obtundation, daytime sedation, balance disturbances, etc., with the addition of any central nervous system depressant, especially in the frail elderly; close monitoring and low-dose titration are important.

1. Insomnia-specific hypnotic agents
   a. Zolpidem 2.5 to 5 mg PO HS, titrate up to 10 mg as needed/tolerated
   CAUTION: very rapid onset
   b. Remelteon 8 mg PO HS

NOTE: this is a relatively new agent that is unique in its mechanism of action, (melatonin receptor agonist) and has very few drug-drug interactions-a notable exception is that it is contraindicated with concurrent use of fluvoxamine.

2. Benzodiazapines
   a. Lorazapam 0.5 to 1 mg PO HS
   b. Temazepam 15 to 30 mg PO HS
3. Sedating antidepressants
   a. Trazadone 25 to 50 mg PO HS, titrate upward as needed
   b. Amitriptyline or doxepin 10 to 25 mg PO HS, titrate upward as needed and as tolerated, monitoring anticholinergic effects

4. Antihistamines
   a. Diphenhydramine 25 to 50 mg PO HS
   b. Hydroxyzine 12.5 to 25 mg PO HS

NOTE: Paradoxical effects with excitement/agitation/restlessness can occur.

5. Other
   a. Melatonin (available at nutritional supplement stores; be aware of occasional dysphoric effects)
- Initiate pharmacotherapy for nocturnal delirium if nonpharmacological approaches are ineffective:
  1. Neuroleptic agents
     a. Chlorpromazine 25 mg PO HS, titrate upward as needed and tolerated.
     b. Haloperidol 0.5 to 2 mg PO/SQ HS, titrate upward as needed and tolerated.

Psychosocial/Spiritual

- Institute nonpharmacological treatment approaches to anxiety and depression.
- Facilitate discussion and expression of fears and worries.
- Help patient identify and express unresolved issues and spiritual concerns.

Goals/Outcomes

- Normalize patient sleep patterns.
- Relieve distressing nocturnal symptoms.
- Relieve caregiver burden during nocturnal hours.

Documentation in the Medical Record

Initial Assessment

- Sleep patterns and disturbances
- Nocturnal physical/emotional symtpoms
- Medication review

Interdisciplinary Progress Notes

- Identification of contributing factors
- Interventions and results

IDT Care Plan

- Nonpharmacological and pharmacological interventions
- Strategies for caregiver support and contingency plans

Nausea and Vomiting

SITUATION: Recurrent or chronic nausea and/or vomiting

Causes

Biomedical

- Visceral or gastrointestinal tract disorders (e.g., malignancy, bowel obstruction, ileus, constipation)
- Central nervous system disturbances (e.g., neoplasm, increased intracranial pressure)
- Chemical triggers (e.g., odors, tastes, drugs)
- Vestibular disturbances
- Metabolic disturbances (e.g., hypercalcemia, uremia)
- Mechanical triggers (e.g., gagging from coughing, hiccuping, retained secretions)

Psychosocial

- Conditioned response to situational/environmental/emotional/sensory stimuli

Findings

Biomedical

- Continuous or episodic nausea with or without vomiting
- Passive or projectile vomiting independent of or associated with food/fluid or medication intake

Psychosocial

- Varying degrees of withdrawal, fatigue, depressed mood, anxiety, aversion to triggering factors
- Varying degrees of acceptance, frustration, aversion by caregiver

Evaluation

Biomedical

- Systems review and physical examination to assess for:
  - Distention, bloating, evidence of bowel obstruction, peptic ulcer/gastritis/esophagitis, severe constipation or impaction
  - Hepatomegaly
  - Evidence of elevated intracranial pressure (papilledema, headache, altered mental status, spontaneous projectile vomiting)
  - Dehydration
  - Oropharyngeal examination (dentures, thrush, hyperreactive gag reflex)
- Medication review with attention to emetogenic or irritant drugs such as opioids, digoxin, theophylline, chemotherapy agents, NSAIDs
- Frequency, volume, color (e.g., bilious), odor (e.g., feculent), consistency (digested/undigested) of vomitus

- Relationship of nausea/vomiting to any specific recurrent activity, event, position, etc

Psychosocial

- Effect of symptoms on mood, energy, social interaction, interest in activities
- Relationship of symptoms to psychological causes
- Effect of vomiting on caregiver coping

Processes of Care

Practical

- Reduce odors and place visual stimuli that trigger nausea/vomiting out of direct eyesight
- Optimize air circulation
- Have ample supply of fresh cold water for mouth rinsing and to apply to the back of the neck and brow
- Institute appropriate level of care in order to implement indicated symptom management and support
- Minimize oral intake to the degree preferred by the patient; reinstitute clear liquids as desired after 24 hours of relief from vomiting. Discontinue all oral intake if bowel obstruction is suspected or confirmed

Biomedical

- Basic principles
  1. Obviate and treat the underlying cause whenever possible
  2. Prevention is more successful than treatment
  3. Use nonpharmacological approaches whenever possible
  4. The oral route is preferred for prophylactic pharmacotherapy
  5. Use the rectal or parenteral (e.g., subcutaneous) route to initiate treatment for the first 24 to 48 hours to control symptoms; then convert to the oral route if possible
  6. Use combination therapies of mechanistically different agents without similar toxicities for intractable symptoms
- Pharmacotherapy for nausea/vomiting due to:
  1. Delayed gastric emptying
     a. Metoclopramide 10 to 20 mg PO q6-8hr; 1 to 2 mg/hr SQ infusion
     b. Add simethicone/charcoal to decrease gas, if eructation is present.
     c. Decrease intrinsic and extrinsic abdominal pressure: elevate head of bed, use loose-fitting and nonbinding clothing
  2. Initiation or escalation of opioid therapy
     a. Metoclopramide 10 to 20 mg PO q6-8hr; 1 to 2 mg/hr SQ infusion
     b. Diphenhydramine 25 to 50 mg PO q6-8hr
     c. Prochlorperazine 25 mg PR or trimethobenzamide 200 mg PR q6hr

- Reassess in 3 to 4 days; tolerance to nausea and emetogenic effects of opioids usually occurs, allowing discontinuation of these antiemetic drugs; If nausea and/or vomiting continue(s), assess for other causes prior to changing analgesic
  3. Bowel obstruction (nonsurgical care in terminal stage of disease)
     a. Octreotide 150 µg IM q12hr or 300 µg/24 hr continuous SQ infusion, combined with opioid analgesic, titrated to effect
     b. Nasogastric suctioning only if necessary, feasible, and tolerated
  4. Vestibular disturbance
     o Meclizine 25 mg bid
  5. Vagal stimulation (bowel obstruction, hepatic capsular pressure, thrush)
     o Scopolamine 0.3 to 0.6 mg SQ prn (monitor for psychotomimetic effects)
  6. Increased intracranial pressure (brain tumor or metastasis)
     o Dexamethasone 4 mg q8hr and increase as necessary to control symptoms
  7. Metabolic abnormalities (hypercalcemia, uremia)
     o Haloperidol 0.5 mg q6-8hr
- Nonspecific and adjunctive therapy
  1. The use of dopamine receptor antagonists (e.g., haloperidol 0.5 to 2 mg PO/IV q6hr prn or prochlorperazine 10 to 25 mg PO/25 to 100 mg PR q6hr prn) in patients who can tolerate the sedating effects is generally effective as primary or adjunctive therapy for most causes of severe nausea and vomiting. These agents are contraindicated in patients with Parkinson's disease.
  2. The addition of lorazapam 0.5 to 2 mg SL/IV may be useful as an adjunctive agent for control of nausea associated with many etiologies, or when there are nonspecified causes.
  3. Dexamethasone is frequently used in the prevention and treatment of chemotherapy and radiation therapy induced nausea and vomiting, as an adjunctive therapy with dopamine receptor antagonists, benzodiazapines, and/or serotonin (5-HT)$_3$ receptor blockers (see below).
  4. Ondansetron (4 to 8 mg IV/PO q6-12hr), granisetron (1 to 2 mg PO q12hr [available as tablets and oral solution 1 mg/5 ml] or 10 µg/kg), and dolasetron (100 mg PO or 1.8 mg/kg IV) are 5-HT$_3$ receptor blockers that have been used for control of nausea and vomiting associated with chemotherapy and certain postoperative circumstances. The newest of these agents, palonosetron is the most potent, and is recommended only as a single 0.25 mg IV dose. These drugs should be considered in those cases resistant to therapies listed earlier.
  5. Aprepitant (125 mg PO followed by 80 mg PO QD) is a substance P antagonist and may be used in conjunction with other antiemetics for refractory nausea/vomiting resulting from oncological therapies.

Psychosocial

- Use imaging and relaxation techniques to control anxiety or apprehension associated with or causing nausea/vomiting
- Teach caregiver management techniques to minimize stress and burden to the extent possible

Goals/Outcomes

- Minimize nausea
- Decrease episodes of vomiting to a maximum of one or two episodes per day
- Reduce care burden
- Reduce social isolation brought on by intractable nausea and vomiting

Documentation in the Medical Record

Initial Assessment

- Frequency and characteristics of nausea/vomiting episodes
- Likely etiology and/or associated causative factors
- Nutritional/hydration status
- Emotional/psychological status: mood, sleep, social interaction, energy
- Physical findings: oropharyngeal and abdominal examination, skin turgor, activity level
- Coping ability of caregiver around this symptom complex

Interdisciplinary Progress Notes

- Description, sequence, and timing of interventions attempted
- Results of interventions, including adverse effects (if any) of pharmacotherapy
- Emotional and physical findings from follow-up visits; caregiver capabilities and coping

IDT Care Plan

- Timing, sequence, and types of interventions
- Schedule of follow-up visits and contingency plans

Pain

SITUATION: Continuous and/or intermittant pain that interferes with basic functions, activities, sleep, social interaction, or otherwise erodes the patient's quality of life to any meaningful extent

Pain is a very common symptom in cancer and other chronic progressive disease states. Along with severe anxiety/agitation and dyspnea, pain that is out of control represents one of the urgent-emergent symptom complexes encountered in the hospice setting. Pain assessment, establishment of patient goals, and intervention plans should be put into place as a high priority. Rapid responses of the team to calls for help when pain is out of control and the abiltity to intervene effectively in a timely manner are key and fundamental measures of quality hospice care.

All hospice practitioners should be familiar with the basic principles of pain assessment and management, as elaborated in Miaskowski C, Cleary J, Burney R, et al. Guideline for the Management of Cancer Pain in Adults and Children. APS Clinical Practice Guidelines Series, No. 3. Glenview, IL, 2005, American Pain Society.

Causes

Biomedical

- Basic principle: Identify the cause of pain, and treat with the most appropriate intervention.
    1. Cancer related: Pain associated with direct or metastatic tumor involvement of bone, nerves, viscera, or soft tissues (60% to 80% of all cancer patients)
    2. Treatment related:
        a. Pain associated with antineoplastic therapy (20% to 25% of cancer patients) such as surgery, radiation therapy and chemotherapy
        b. Pain caused by noncancer drug therapy or surgery
    3. Other common painful disorders associated with advanced disease states:
        a. Myofascial pain (muscle trigger point pain with radiating and referred pain)
        b. Arthropathies (joint pains most commonly due to osteoarthritis, degenerative joint disease, or rheumatoid arthritis)
        c. Neuropathies (e.g., diabetes, peripheral vascular disease, herpes zoster)
        d. Headache (tension pattern, migraine, mixed, other)
        e. Skin and mucosal ulceration
        f. Constipation
        g. Back pain (spinal stenosis, facet disease, spondylosis/disc disease, other)

Psychosocial/Spiritual

- Basic principle: Any amount of pain can lead to a lot of suffering, and any amount of suffering can greatly amplify the pain experience.
    1. Pain due to any disease is often greatly amplified by interpersonal conflict or unresolved intrapersonal issues (psychological or spiritual), especially when the pain is a constant reminder of the seriousness of the illness
    2. Pain, anxiety, and depression reinforce each other as complex psychophysiological interactions that oftentimes cannot be readily separated; Detailed assessment is necessary in order to direct therapy in the most specific and efficacious way;

Findings

Biomedical

- Patient report of pain/discomfort
- Facial expressions or body posturing suggestive of pain, e.g., grimacing, guarding
- Vocalizations suggestive of pain
- Tachycardia, tachypnea, hypertension, diaphoresis

NOTE: Absence of these autonomic findings do not rule out pain; presence of these findings in a noncommunicating patient is suggestive, especially when repositioning.

Psychosocial

- Poor sleep
- Decreased coping
- Agitation/restlessness
- Withdrawal from social interaction
- Decreased interest in previous enjoyments, e.g., television viweing, reading, sewing, life review
- Signs/symptoms of depression, anxiety

Evaluation (see Figure 3.1)

Biomedical and Psychosocial/Spiritual

- Basic principle: Believe the patient's report of pain. Because pain is a subjective phenomenon, the caregiver/clinician must believe the patient's report of pain is real; Objective physiological indicators of acute pain such as tachycardia, sweating, pallor, or affective responses such as facial grimacing are helpful when present but are often absent when pain is chronic or continuous
- Take a careful history including:
  1. Onset (When did it/does it start?)
  2. Duration (How long does it last?)
  3. Location (Where does it start, and where does it spread?)
  4. Quality (e.g., burning, aching, etc.)
  5. Pain gets worse with . . .
  6. Pain gets better with . . .
  7. Pain intensity (measure in able patients using patient's pain rating): measure and record using a standard rating scale (see Figure 3.2: make copies for patient as needed)
     a. Present pain
     b. Average continuous pain throughout the day
     c. Breakthrough pain: frequency, severity, and duration
        o Incident pain (caused by specific activity or action)
        o Spontaneous pain (no identifiable cause)
        o End-of-dose failure (pain returns before next dose of regularly scheduled medicine takes effect)

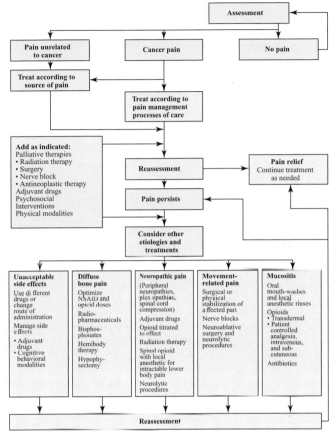

Figure 3.1 Flow Chart for continuing evaluation and treatment of pain (Adapted from AHCPR Clinical Guideline Number 9).

8. Use of a 24-hour pain diary in an able patient helps to identify many factors and effects of interventions (see Figure 3.3: make copies for patient/caregiver as needed)

- Assess the effect of pain on the patient's mood, ADLs, sleep, appetite, movement, toileting, social interactions, interest in life, and previous enjoyments
- Take a careful analgesic history including prior and present medications, analgesic response (time to onset of meaningful pain relief and duration of action), and undesirable or adverse effects, including frank allergies and gastrointestinal upset

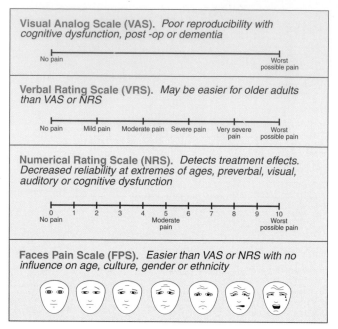

Figure 3.2 Unidimensional Pain Scale [reprinted from the Journal of Pain, May;41(2). Bieri D, Reeve RA, Champion GD, Addicoat L, Ziegler JB. The Faces Pain Scale for the self-assessment of the severity of pain experienced by children: Development, initial validation, and preliminary investigation for ratio scale properties, pp 139–150, ©1990 with permission from Elsevier).

- Perform physical examination and review systems specific to pain complaints.
- Review and consider necessity for corroborating diagnostic testing *only* in cases where diagnosis is in question or treatment/care plan will be meaningfully effected (e.g., radiograph for suspected pathological fracture)
- Treat pain empirically while evaluation is being completed
- Be as specific as possible in determining the cause of the pain whenever possible (e.g., fecal impaction, bowel obstruction, epidural metastasis, plexopathy, lytic bone lesion, etc.) and institute diagnosis-specific therapy immediately
- Evaluate level of anxiety and signs of depressive mood disorder
- Evaluate for contributors to pain/suffering of a psychological/spiritual nature, e.g., guilt, punishment, abandonment by God, etc
- Evaluate patient/caregiver understanding and use of nonpharmacological pain reducing interventions (e.g., relaxation, imaging, meditation, music, massage, heat, cooling, etc.)
- Reevaluate pain complaints and effects of interventions frequently

Twenty-four Hour Pain Diary

Patient Name: _____ Date: _____

Time	Maximal Pain 0-10 scale	Minimal Pain 0-10 scale	Medication: name, dose, route of administration	Activities: lying, sitting, walking, eating, toilet, etc.
12 Midnight				
1 am				
2				
3				
4				
5				
6				
7				
8				
9				
10				
11				
12 Noon				
1 pm				
2				
3				
4				
5				
6				
7				
8				
9				
10				
11				

Figure 3.3 Twenty-four hour pain diary.

- Determine appropriate level of care, based on patient/caregiver response to therapies and coping abilities.

Processes of Care

Biomedical (see Figures 3.4 and 3.5)

- Basic principles of pain management
  - o Use the least invasive and most readily available and acceptable (to the patient/caregiver) agent/route of administration possible. This is usually the oral route
  - o Administer analgesics on a regularly scheduled basis, "around-the-clock" (ATC), rather than "prn" for continuous pain problems. Sustained or continuous release formulations make this easier.

o Treat breakthrough pain.
- MODERATE-SEVERE PAIN TREATMENT PROTOCOL: Analgesic dose titration for pain that is out of control
  1. Initiate pain treatment protocol within 1 hour for residential/home patients and within 15 minutes for inpatients
  2. Immediately reassess and determine cause of pain.
  3. Administer breakthrough pain dose of ordered analgesic; repeat in 15 to 30 minutes if ineffective at bringing pain under control.
  4. If pain still poorly controlled, increase breakthrough pain analgesic dose by 50% to 100%.
  5. **If pain is well controlled**, increase baseline (around the clock) dose of analgesic by 50% and continue with newly adjusted breakthrough pain analgesic.
     a. Reassess in 24 hours and adjust medication dose based on patient's clinical status.
     b. Adjust bowel regimen accordingly.
  6. **If pain continues out of control** (by patient report of pain out of control or behavior suggestive of uncontrolled pain in noncommunicative patient) 4 hours after initiating protocol, repeat steps 1 through 4 and notify on-call physician;
  7. If no significant improvement in pain control 8 hours after initiating protocol, discuss with physician and consider pain management consultation.
  8. If patient is in imminent dying phase, institute pain crisis protocol (see later); notify physician of clinical circumstances.

Pharmacotherapy (see Table 3.1)

  1. NSAIDs and acetaminophen
     a. Indications/advantages
        o Mild to moderate pain
        o Inflammatory pain syndromes, including bone pain
        o Minimal effect on mental functioning
        o Supplement with opioid analgesics for moderate to severe pain
        o Available over-the-counter in a variety of forms
        o Coxibs (COX-2 selective NSAIDs) do not affect platelet adhesion and so are preferred over nonselective NSAIDs when there is a risk of bleeding or patients have thrombocytopenia. Short-term use is associated with less gastrointestinal risk.
     b. Contraindications/disadvantages
        o Gastrointestinal distress and ulceration (nonselective NSAIDs)
        o Platelet dysfunction/bleeding (nonselective NSAIDs)
        o Hypersensitivity reactions (NSAIDs)
        o Hepatic/renal impairment (NSAIDs and acetaminophen)
  2. Opioid Analgesics (see Table 3.2, a and b)
- Indications: Moderate to severe pain

		3rd Line Refractory Pain or Dose-Limiting Side Effects
	2nd Line Moderate to Severe Pain or Pain Out of Control	Spinal Opioids $\pm\alpha_2$-adrenergic agonist $\pm$ local anesthetic
1st Line Mild to Moderate Pain	Opioids NSAIDs Pain Modulators*	Nerve Block Neurolysis/Ablation Neurostimulation Total Analgesia Subanesthetic ketamine IV local anesthetic Total Sedation e.g., Propofol, Etomidate,
Acetaminophen NSAIDs Pain Modulators*		

* e.g., anticonvulsants, tricyclic and serotonin/norepinephrine reuptake inhibitor antidepressants, corticosteroids, local anesthetics, α_2-adrenergic agonists.

Figure 3.4 Modification of World Health Organization Step Ladder Approach to Pain Control (reprinted with permission from Fine PG. The evolving and important role of anesthesiology in palliative care. Anesth Analg 2005;100:183–188 with permission from Lippincott, Williams and Wilkins.)

- Contraindications: Allergy
- Precautions: Use of agonist-antagonist drugs contraindicated (pentazocine; butorphanol; nalbuphine). Meperidine use discouraged due to toxic metabolite (normeperidine). Intramuscular use highly discouraged except in "pain emergency" states while other routes are being established or transdermal drugs are being titrated. The oral transmucosal route for rapid delivery of fentanyl may obviate the necessity to ever use the intramuscular route for pain control. Anticipate, prevent, and treat sedation, constipation, nausea, psychotomimetic effects, respiratory depression, and myoclonus.
- Dose conversions: Changing from one opioid to another, or one route to another, is often necessary and facility with this process is an absolute necessity. Triple check your calculations and ask a colleague to check your conclusions if there is any question. Remember the following points:
  - Incomplete cross-tolerance occurs, leading to decreased requirements of a newly prescribed agent.
  - Use morphine parenteral equivalents as a "common denominator" for all dose conversions in order to avoid errors.
- Opioid analgesics: Specific features, caveats, cautions, and quirks

Table 3.1 Acetaminophen and a Selection of Over-the-Counter and Prescription Nonsteroidal Anti-inflammatory Drugs

Drug	>50-kg Dose	<50-kg Dose
Acetaminophen*†	4000 mg/24 hr	10-15 mg/kg q4hr (oral)
	(q4-6hr dosing)	15-20 mg/hg q4hr (rectal)
Aspirin*†	4000 mg/24 hr	10-15 mg/kg q4hr (oral)
	(q4-6hr dosing)	15-20 mg/kg q4hr (rectal)
Ibuprofen*†	2400 mg/24 hr	10 mg/kg q6-8hr (oral)
	(q6-8hr dosing)	
Naproxen*†	1000 mg/24 hr	5 mg/kg q8hr (oral/rectal)
	(q8-12hr dosing)	
Choline magnesium	5500 mg/24 hr	25 mg/kg q8hr (oral)
trisalicylate*‡	(q8-12hr dosing)	
Celecoxib‡§	200 mg/24 hr (q12-24hr dosing)	3 mg/kg/24 hr (max 200 mg)
Ketorolac	30-60 mg IM/IV initially, then 15-30 mg q6hr bolus IV/IM or continuous IV/SQ infusion; SHORT-TERM USE ONLY	

*Commercially available in a liquid form.

†Commercially available in a suppository form.

‡Minimal effect on platelet function (preferred to nonselective and acetylating NSAIDs in patients subject to bleeding or thrombocytopenia).

§Reduced GI adverse effects compared with nonselective NSAIDS with short-term or intermittent use.

Table 3.2a. Approximate Equianalgesic Doses of Most Commonly Recommended Opioid Analgesics*

Drug	Parenteral Dose	Enteral Dose
Morphine (1)	10 mg	30 mg
Codeine	130 mg	200 mg
Fentanyl (2)	50 to 100 μg	
Hydrocodone		30 mg
Hydromorphone	1.5 mg	7.5 mg
Levorphanol (3)	2 mg	4 mg
Methadone (3)	See Table 3.2b	
Oxycodone (4)		20 to 30 mg
Oxymorphone (5)	1 mg	10 mg

*Dose conversion should be closely monitored because incomplete cross-tolerance may occur.

(1) Available in continuous and sustained release formulations lasting 8 to 24 hours.

(2) Also available in both transdermal and oral transmucosal forms.

(3) These drugs have long and variable half-lives so accumulation can occur; close monitoring during first few days of therapy is very important.

(4) Available in several continuous release doses that last 8 to 12 hours.

(5) Available as immediate (q4-6hr) and extended release (q12hr dosing) formulations.

Table 3.2b. Dosing Guidelines for Oral Methadone

Daily Oral Morphine Dose Equivalents	Conversion Ratio of Oral Morphine to Oral Methadone
<100 mg	3:1 (i.e., 3 mg morphine:1 mg methadone)
101 to 300 mg	5:1
301 to 600 mg	10:1
601 to 800 mg	12:1
801 to 1000 mg	15:1
>1000 mg	20:1

Due to incomplete cross-tolerance and variable potency, it is recommended that when switching to methadone, the initial dose is 50% to 75% of the equianalgesic dose, but be prepared to provide rescue doses of an immediate-acting short half-life opioid (e.g., morphine, hydrocodone, oxycodone, hydromorphone) while achieving steady-state doses of methadone (up to 5 to 7 days of tid dosing).

Morphine

- Most often considered the "gold standard" of opioid analgesics.
- Some patients cannot tolerate morphine due to itching, headache, dysphoria, or other adverse effects.
- The metabolites of morphine (morphine-3-glucuronide and morphine-6-glucuronide) may contribute to sedation, myoclonus, and psychotomimetic effects.
- Common effects such as sedation and nausea often resolve within a few days.
- Convert to an equianalgesic dose of a different opioid if adverse effects exceed benefit.
- Anticipate adverse effects, especially constipation, nausea, and sedation, and prevent or treat appropriately.
- Oral morphine solution can be swallowed or small volumes (½ to 1 ml) of a concentrated solution (e.g., 20 mg/ml) can be placed under the tongue for partial mucosal absorption into the bloodstream, although most of the effect is obtained by enteral absorption after swallowing.
- Morphine's bitter taste may be prohibitive in unflavored forms, especially if "immediate release" tablets are left in the mouth to dissolve.
- Nebulized morphine has been reported to relieve dyspnea (air hunger) in some patients. Whether this is due to systemic uptake or due to specific interactions between the drug and receptors within the lower respiratory tract is not yet known. Initial dose recommendation: 2 to 4 mg "injectable" or preservative-free MS in 2.5 ml saline for nebulization.

Fentanyl

- Transdermal fentanyl (fentanyl patch): Opioid-naive patients should start with a 25 µg/hr patch and be very closely observed for the first 24 to 48 hours of therapy until steady-state blood levels are attained. Use 12-hour oral morphine equivalent dose to convert to microgram per hour dose size of patch: e.g., for a patient using 100 mg oral morphine every 12 hours, use a 100 μg/hr fentanyl patch. Time to peak and steady state blood levels for patients starting the patch is usually 18 to 24 hours. Make sure other rapid-onset dosage forms of an opioid analgesic are available during this time period and for breakthrough pains later on. Although the currently available fentanyl patch is formulated for 72-hour use, end-of-dose failure often occurs as early as 48 hours. Close monitoring of efficacy, duration of effect, breakthrough pain episodes and medication use, and adverse effects is important during the first several days of use and during periods of advancing disease with increasing pain, until a stable pattern of effectiveness is reached.

Instructions to Patients
1. Place patch on the upper body in a clean, dry, hairless area.
2. Choose a different site when placing a new patch, then remove the old patch.
3. Remove the old patch or patches and fold sticky surfaces together, then flush down the toilet.
4. Wash hands after handling patches.
5. All unused patches (patient discontinued use or deceased) should be removed from wrappers, folded in half with sticky surfaces together, and flushed down the toilet.
    o Oral transmucosal fentanyl citrate (OTFC): For adults, start with the 200 μg dose for breakthrough pain, and monitor efficacy, advancing to higher dose units as needed. Onset of pain relief can usually be expected in about 5 minutes after beginning use. Any remaining partial units should be disposed of safely by placing under hot water or clipping the unused medication off of the stick and flushing down the toilet.

Hydromorphone
- Hydromorphone is 5 to 8 times more potent than morphine, permitting analgesic equivalence at lower doses and smaller volumes
- Hydromorphone can be administered through oral, parenteral (subcutaneous, intramuscular, and intravenous), rectal, or intraspinal (epidural and intrathecal) routes
- Hydromorphone's relatively short half-life of elimination (2 to 3 hours) facilitates dose titration.Onset of action occurs within 15 minutes after parenteral administration and within 30 minutes after oral or rectal administration
- Since hydromorphone is highly soluble in water (about 300 mg/ml), it is particularly suitable for subcutaneous administration, including continuous subcutaneous infusion (CSCI) and patient-controlled analgesia (PCA).
- Hydromorphone is hydrophilic and extensively distributes in the cerebral spinal fluid (CSF) on epidural administration

- A high-potency preparation (10 mg/ml) is commercially available for opioid-tolerant patients. This preparation is particularly useful for CSCI in patients where small volumes are necessary
- Side effects associated with hydromorphone are qualitatively similar to those associated with opioids in general and most often include constipation, nausea, and sedation; Hydromorphone may be preferred in patients with decreased renal clearance in order to prevent toxic metabolite accumulation associated with other morphine.

Levorphanol and Methadone

- These drugs are useful in selected patients as time-contingent analgesics due to their long biological half-lives, making dosing intervals (q6-8hr) relatively convenient; The potential for drug accumulation prior to achievement of steady-state blood levels (4 to 6 doses) puts patients at risk for oversedation and respiratory depression; Close monitoring for these potentially adverse effects is required by an observant caregiver; Recent evidence suggests that even low doses of methadone may put patients at risk for arrhythmias due to prolongation of the QT (repolarization) interval; Caution needs to be exercised in patients with electrolyte abnormalities, cardiac conduction abnormalities, and when escalating doses of the drug

Sustained or Continuous Release Enteral Formulations

- Several opioids are now available in sustained or continuous release form, facilitating compliance and maintaining blood levels between dosing intervals for improved overall control of continuous types of pain
- Morphine: Commercially available continuous release pill formulations of morphine last 8 to 24 hours. The continuous release formulations have similar effects when administered rectally, applied with a small amount of water-based lubricant to ease insertion (no encapsulation is necessary). A sustained release morphine formulation of pellets in a capsule is available that lasts up to 24 hours but cannot be used per rectum; The capsules can be opened and the contents sprinkled on to a palatable food (e.g., apple sauce) as an alternative to swallowing them whole
- Oxycodone: Continuous release oxycodone lasts 8 to 12 hours and is available in several dose sizes, starting at 10 mg
- Oxymorphone: continuous release oxymorphone lasts 12 hours and is available in several dose sizes, starting with 5 mg

  NOTE: Chewing or crushing continuous release formulations causes them to be IMMEDIATE RELEASE, potentially subjecting the patient to overdosage.

Preventing and Treating Opioid Adverse Effects

- Constipation: Always begin a prophylactic bowel regimen when commencing opioid analgesic therapy

- o Avoid bulking agents (e.g., psyllium) because these tend to cause a larger, bulkier stool, increasing dessication time in the large bowel
- o Encourage fluid (fruit juice) intake
- o Encourage dietary regimens (use of Senna tea and fruits)
- o For pharmacotherapy, refer to previous section on constipation

- Excessive sedation: After dose titration for appropriate pain control, and other correctable causes have been identified and treated if possible, use of psychostimulants may be beneficial
  - o Dextroamphetamine 2.5 to 5 mg PO every morning and mid-day
  - o Methylphenidate 5 to 10 mg PO every morning and 2.5 to 5 mg midday
  - o Adjust both dose and timing to prevent nocturnal insomnia
  - o Monitor for undesirable psychotomimetic effects (agitation, hallucinations, irritability)
  - o Modafinil 100 to 200 mg PO every morning. This is a relatively safe and effective central nervous system stimulant that is well tolerated in most patients, but it is relatively expensive

- Respiratory depression: This is rarely a clinically significant problem for opioid tolerant patients in pain. When undesired depressed consciousness occurs along with a respiratory rate <8/min or hypoxemia (O_2 saturation <90%) associated with opioid use, cautious and slow titration of naloxone should be instituted; Excessive administration may cause abrupt opioid reversal with pain and autonomic crisis. Dilute 1 ampule of naloxone (0.4 mg/ml) 1:10 in injectable saline (final concentration 40 μg/ml) and inject 1 ml every 2 to 3 minutes while closely monitoring level of consciousness and respiratory rate

- Nausea/vomiting: Common with opioids, but habituation occurs in most cases within several days. Assess for other treatable causes; Doses of antiemetics as follows are initial doses, which can be increased as required
  - o Metoclopramide 10 mg PO/IV q6hr
  - o Diphenhydramine 25 mg PO/IV q6hr
  - o Prochlorperazine 25 to 50 mg PO/PR q6hr
  - o Promethazine 25 to 50 mg PO/PR q6hr
  - o Haloperidol 0.5 mg IV q6hr or 2 mg PO q6hr
  - o Droperidol ¼ to ½ ml IV q6hr
  - o Ondansetron 4 mg PO/IV q8hr

- Myoclonus: occurs more commonly with high-dose opioid therapy; Use of an alternate drug is recommended, especially if using morphine, due to metabolite accumulation; A lower dose of the substitute drug may be possible due to incomplete cross-tolerance
  - o Clonazepam 0.5 mg PO q6-8hr may be useful in treating myoclonus in patients who are still alert and able to communicate and take oral preparations; Increase as needed and tolerated

- o Diazepam 2 to 5 mg IV as needed to control myoclonus in imminently dying patients with intravenous access may be helpful.
- Pruritus: Most common with morphine, thought to be due to histamine release, but can occur with most opioids. Treatment-induced sedation must be viewed by the patient as an acceptable tradeoff.
  1. Antihistamines
     - o Diphenhydramine 25 to 50 mg PO/IV q6hr
     - o Hydroxyzine 25 mg PO q6hr
  2. Benzodiazepines
     - o Lorazepam 1 mg SL/PO/IV q6hr

Pain-Modulating Drugs ("Adjuvant Analgesics") (see Table 3.3)

Basic principle: Always consider the addition of pain modulating agents when there is a specific pathophysiological indication (e.g., bone pain; neuropathic pain), when there is inadequate pain control with primary analgesic therapy alone, when there is sleep disturbance, or when opioid adverse effects predominate.

- Pain crises: The first approach to treating pain that has increased beyond the patient's level of comfort is to methodically evaluate the cause, in order to determine the most therapeutically specific means to treat it, while ensuring comfort as quickly and effectively as possible. Table 3.5 outlines a basic approach to immediate analgesic treatment for patients taking around-the-clock opioid analgesics. The on-call physician and IDT should be notified as soon as possible throughout all phases of treatment to ensure that the most appropriate comprehensive care plan is considered and actualized. The patient's primary care physician or referring physician should be notified in a timely manner, depending on her/his specifications regarding ongoing communication of patient status.
- Most somatic and visceral pain is controllable with appropriately administered analgesic therapy. Some neuropathic pains, e.g., invasive and compressive neuropathies, plexopathies, and myelopathies, may be poorly responsive to analgesic therapies, short of inducing a nearly comatose state. Widespread bone metastases or end-stage pathological fractures may present similar challenges.
- Differentiate terminal agitation or anxiety from "physically" based pain, if possible. Terminal symptoms unresponsive to rapid upward titration of opioid may respond to benzodiazepines (e.g., diazepam; lorazepam; refer to "Agitation and Anxiety" and "Imminent Death").
- Make sure drugs are getting absorbed. The only *guaranteed* route is the intravenous route; Although this is to be avoided unless necessary, if there is any question about absorption of analgesics, parenteral access should be established
- Preterminal pain crises that are poorly responsive to basic approaches to analgesic therapy merit consultation with a pain management consultant as

Table 3.3. Pain-Modulating Drugs

| | DAILY ADULT STARTING DOSE | | |
Drug	Dose Range	Route(s) of Administration	Indications
Corticosteroids			Cerebral edema, spinal cord compression, bone pain, neuropathic pain
Dxamethasone	2 to 4 mg tid-qid	PO/IV/SQ	
Prednisone	15 to 30 mg tid-qid	PO	
Tricyclic antidepressants	10 to 25 mg hs	PO	Neuropathic pain, sleep disturbance
Amitriptyline			
Desipramine			
Imipramine			
Nortriptyline			
Doxepin			
Anticonvulsants			Neuropathic pain
Clonazapam	0.5 to 1 mg hs-bid-tid	PO	
Carbamazapine	100 mg qd-tid	PO	
Gagabapentin	100 mg qd-tid	PO	
Pregabalin	25 to 50 mg qd (titritate to bid-tid dosing)	PO	
Local Anesthetics			Neuropathic pain
Mexiletine	150 mg qd-tid	PO	
Lidocaine	10 to 25 mg/hr	IV or SQ infusion	
Lidocaine 5% transdermal patch: apply to healthy skin overlying painful areas			
Bisphosphonates (see Table 3.4)			
Calcium channel blockers			
Nifedipine	10 mg tid	PO	Ischemic pain,
			neuropathic pain, smooth muscle
			spasms with pain

quickly as possible; Radiotherapy, anesthetic, or neuroablative procedures may be indicated

- Consider spinal/epidural opioid/local anesthetic approaches, neurolytic celiac plexus block, or spinothalamic tractotomy. Expertise in these techniques is required; credentials AND experience should be determined in advance of referral.

- From a case-management standpoint, these interventions can add greatly to quality of life and decrease costs if a patient's pain is inadequately controlled by appropriate dose titration of opioid analgesics and adjuvants

- For truly intractable end-stage pain, parenteral administration of ketamine will provide relief for the patient, and ease the great distress that witnessing

Table 3.4. Comparison of Commonly Used Parenteral and Newer Oral Bisphosphonates in Cancer Patients With Metastatic Bone Disease

Bisphosphonate Generic Name (Brand Name)	Efficacy in Metastatic Bone Disease	Formulations	Effective Dose	Price* (monthly cost)
ibandronate† (Boniva)	Effective by oral and IV routes	IV	6 mg infusion over 1 to 2 hours q3-4weeks	Not available*
		Oral (2.5 mg tablet)	50 mg/day	Not available*
pamidronate‡ (Aredia)	Oral route not effective in multiple myeloma or breast cancer; IV route is effective	IV (3 mg/ml, 10 ml vial and 9 mg/ml, 10 ml vial)	90 mg infusion over 2 hours q3-4weeks	$870.00
zoledronic acid‡ (Zometa)	IV route very effective, but no oral preparation available	4 mg/5 ml 5 ml vial	4 mg infusion over 15 minutes q4weeks	$959.41

*AWP. Redbook, 2004. Thompson Healthcare, Bethesda, MD. Cost per treatment varies with treatment length.

While AWP prices may provide a relative cost, it is important to consider other contributors to overall cost when using bisphosphonates for metastatic disease. Nursing staff cost of IV equipment and preparation if using IV preparation, hospital admission time, and adverse events that may occur, etc. It is important to individualize cost when comparing agents, but oral bisphosphonates, such as ibandronate, offer a large advantage over IV preparations due no real need for supportive personnel, additional equipment and facility charges.

Oral and intravenous formulations approved in Europe for breast cancer patients with bone metastases.

‡Approved in the United States and recommended by the American Society of Clinical Oncologists (ASCO) for treatment of breast cancer patients with bone metastases. Best results have been demonstrated with zoledronic acid.

such agony can cause family and other caregivers who need or want to remain in attendance.

o BOLUS: Ketamine 0.1 mg/kg IV. Repeat as often as indicated by the patient's response. Double the dose if no clinical improvement in 5-10 minutes. Follow the bolus with an infusion. Decrease opioid dose by 50%

o INFUSION: Start ketamine at 0.015 mg/kg/min IV (about 1 mg/min for a 70-kg individual). Subcutaneous infusion is possible if IV access is not attainable. In this case, use an initial IM bolus dose of 0.3 to 0.5 mg/kg. Decrease opioid dose by 50%

• It is advisable to administer a benzodiazapine (e.g., diazapam or lorazapam) concurrently to mitigate against the possibility of hallucinations or frightful dreams, since patients under these circumstances may never be able to communicate such experiences

• Observe for problematic increases in secretions; treat with glycopyrrolate, scopalomine, or atropine (see "Imminent Death" section on secretions)

Table 3.5 Analgesic Protocol for Escalating Pain in Opioid-Tolerant Patients

Time (hr)	Treatment
0	Definition of pain out of control: Continuous pain > 4 to 5/10 not responsive to current analgesic Rx and distressing to patient. 1. Bolus dose (PO, SL, PR, IV, SQ) 50% of equivalent hourly dose with immediate release dose of opioid analgesic and 2. Increase ATC doses 50% (notify physician and rest of IDT as soon as time allows).
1	3. If pain still out of control after 1 hour, rebolus as per No. 1.
2	4. If no appreciable change, notify physician for further orders.
3 to 4	5. If recommendations by hospice/primary care physician(s) do not lead to adequate pain control (pain continues >4 to 5/10 and distressing to patient): *Recommend*: 1) opioid rotation; i.e., equivalent dose of alternative opioid analgesic. 2) Parenteral opioid administration (if not already route of administration) with dose titration at bedside.
6 to 8	6. If pain continues out of control, contact medical director 7. Consider continuous care versus general inpatient care. 8. Review indications for other approaches to pain control.

Breakthrough Pain: Intermittent Episodes of Moderate to More Severe Pain That Occurs Despite Control of Baseline Continuous Pains Are Very Common (see Fig. 3.5)

Although best studied in cancer patients, there is evidence that patients with other pain-producing, life-limiting diseases experience breakthrough pain a few times a day, lasting moments to many minutes. The risk of increasing the ATC analgesic dose is increasing adverse effects, especially sedation, once the more short-lived, episodic breakthrough pain has remitted.

1. Subtypes and treatment
   a. Incident pain: Pain that is predictably elicited by specific activities. Use a rapid-onset, short-duration analgesic formulation in anticipation of pain-eliciting activities or events. Adjust dose to severity of anticipated pain or the intensity/duration of the pain-producing event. Past experience will serve as the best guide.
   b. Spontaneous pain: Unpredictable pain, not temporally associated with any activity or event. These pains are more challenging to control. Use of adjuvants for neuropathic pains may help diminish frequency and severity of these types of pains (see Table 3.3). Otherwise, immediate treatment with a potent, rapid-onset opioid analgesic is indicated:
      o Conventionally, oral morphine solution or other immediate release oral formulations of opioid analgesics have been used most commonly, in order to avoid parenteral administration, but relatively long and inconstant/unpredictable onset times coupled with dura-

tion of effect exceeding the typical breakthrough pain episode limits the utility of this traditional approach.

 o Oral transmucosal fentanyl citrate (OTFC) is an effective, noninvasive means of treating these symptoms. Intravenous bolus dosing for patients with intravenous access may be necessary in those circumstances where oral or transmucosal drugs are not able to be used (PCA devices may be helpful).

c. "End of dose failure" is the phrase used to describe pain that occurs toward the end of the usual dosing interval of a regularly scheduled analgesic. This results from declining blood levels of the ATC analgesic prior to administration or uptake of the next scheduled dose. Appropriate questioning will ensure rapid diagnosis of end of dose failure. Shortening the dose interval to match the onset of this type of breakthrough pain should remedy this problem. For instance, a patient who is taking continuous release morphine every 12 hours whose pain "breaks through" after about 8 to 10 hours is experiencing end of dose failure. The dosing interval should be increased to every 8 hours. If the dose interval becomes too short to make compliance easy, then it is reasonable to increase the dose by 25% to 50%, monitoring closely for therapeutic and adverse effects

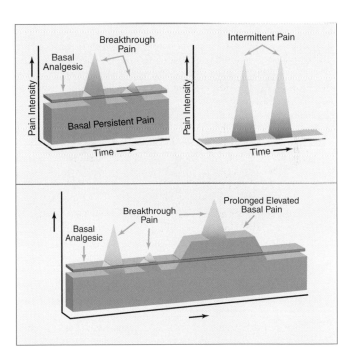

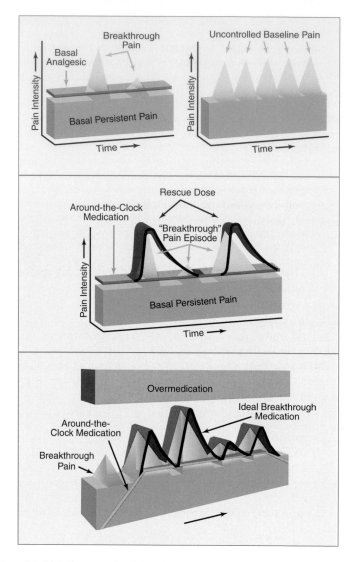

Figure 3.5 (a) Differentiating breakthrough pain from intermittent pain. (b) Differentiating breakthrough pain from prolonged elevated basal pain. (c) Differentiating breakthrough pain from uncontrolled baseline pain. (d) The rescue dose as a conceptual foundation for breakthrough pain.. (e) Management of baseline and breakthrough pain. (All adapted with permission from Fine PG. The Diagnosis and Treatment of Breakthrough Pain. Oxford University Press, New York, 2008).

Goals/Outcomes

- Pain out of control (patient self-report of >3/10 pain, or pain greater than patient's acceptable level) is brought under control within 48 hours of admission to hospice
- Pain out of control is responded to with effective intervention within the prescribed time frames in all patients so that no patient dies with pain out of control
- Analgesic adverse effects and side effects are prevented or effectively managed in all patients

Documentation in the Medical Record

Initial Assessment

- Findings from comprehensive pain assessment
- Current pain management regimen
- Patient/caregiver understanding/expectations/goals of pain management
- Concerns regarding opioids
  - Review of systems pertinent to analgesic use: bowels, balance, memory, etc.

Interdisciplinary Progress Notes

- Ongoing findings from pain reassessment
  - Baseline pain scores
  - Breakthrough pain frequency and severity
  - Effects on function, sleep, activity, social interaction, mood, etc.
- Types and effects (outcomes) of interventions, including adverse effects
- Bowel function, sedation, nausea/vomiting assessments
- Documentation of specific instructions, patient/caregiver understanding, compliance
- Patient/caregiver coping

IDT Care Plan

- Specific pharmacological and nonpharmacological interventions by which members of the IDT
- Contingency plans and crisis prevention/intervention plans reviewed as indicated

Pruritus

SITUATION: Chronic or recurrent itching that impacts negatively on the patient's physical or emotional well-being

Causes

- Overly dry skin (xerosis) and moist skin (maceration) are common and easily treated causes
- Contact dermatitis, drug reactions (allergy), fungal infection, and skin infestations should be considered and either ruled out or treated
- Cholestasis or hepatobiliary disorders are common occurrences in many advanced disease states, due to drug reactions, accumulation of bile salts, or obstruction
- Hodgkin's disease and cutaneous infiltration in malignant diseases cause pruritus
- The majority of patients experiencing chronic renal failure will have this symptom

Findings

- Self-report of itching or behavior suggestive of pruritus in non-communicative patient (e.g., scratching, restlessness)
- Excoriated skin
- Skin rash
- Scratching without relief of symptoms
- Fitful sleep
- Mood alteration (irritability)

Evaluation

- The key to treatment of pruritus (sensation of itching) is identification of the cause. Inadequate treatment can lead to excoriation and secondary infection, sleep deprivation, mood alteration (irritability), and generalized discomfort
- History or symptoms as revealed by patient or observant caregiver
- Identification of likely disease-related causes
- Physical examination of the skin
- Identification of environmental-related causes

Processes of Care

- For xerosis or macerated skin, use lubricating or drying techniques and materials, respectively
- Nonspecific pharmacotherapy can be used until specific treatments take effect or as an adjunct if adequate resolution does not occur

1. Sedating agents with some antihistamine activity, especially at night, will promote rest and sleep. Titrate choice of drug slowly, monitory therapeutic effects versus undesirable side effects:
   a. Hydroxyzine (25 to 50 mg PO q6hr)
   b. Doxepin (10 to 50 mg PO HS)
   c. Promethazine (25 to 50 mg IV q4-6hr)
   d. Diphenhydramine (25 to 50 PO/IV q6hr)
   e. Cyproheptadine (pediatrics: 0.25 mg/kg/day; adults: 0.5 mg/kg/day maximum dose) starting with a low dose and titrating upward, bid to tid PO dosing (syrup = 2 mg/tsp; tablets = 4 mg/tab)
2. Serotonin reuptake inhibitor therapy has been demonstrated to be effective in palliating pruritus not caused by cholestasis or primary dermatological disease:
   o Paroxetine 10 to 30 mg every morning
3. Cholestatic pruritus that is not amenable to drug changes or stenting may respond to salt-binding drugs, such as cholestyramine (4 g PO qid), but this drug is generally not well tolerated in very ill individuals. Palliative medications include:
   a. Maalox 15 ml PO q6hr
   b. Methyltestosterone 25 mg SL bid (caution in hormone-sensitive tumors, except in end-stage symptom control).
   c. Ondansetron 4 to 8 mg (IV/PO) q8-12hr
4. Skin infiltration by malignancies, such as breast cancer, might respond to NSAID therapy, if tolerated. Use maximum anti-inflammatory doses, e.g., naproxen 15 to 20 mg/kg/day in divided doses; ibuprofen 30 to 40 mg/kg/day in divided doses.
5. Opioid-induced pruritus is usually short-lived, with patients becoming rapidly habituated to this effect. Changing to an equally potent dose of another drug (especially a synthetic derivative, because histamine release is common with morphine-like compounds) is one alternative. Use of nonspecific pharmacotherapy as suggested above will generally attenuate symptoms during the habituation phase. Patients with spinal opioid delivery systems may benefit from low-dose naloxone infusion (1 μg/kg/hr) or oral naltrexone (12.5 mg PO daily), slowly increasing the dose as needed.
6. Suspected skin infestation (e.g., scabies) or fungal infection should be treated with the appropriate primary therapy, complemented by nonspecific palliative therapies, as above, to treat symptoms until the cause is effectively treated. Inflammatory skin disorders may respond to topical corticosteroid therapy, e.g., hydrocortisone 0.5% to 1% or triamcinolone acetonide 0.025% cream.

Goals/Outcomes
- Relief of physical and emotional distress associated with pruritus
- Prevention of skin breakdown and infection
- Improved sleep

Documentation in the Medical Record

Initial Assessment

- Severity, location(s), and duration/timing of symptoms
- Aggravating and alleviating factors
- Etiology of symptoms
- Physical examination findings
- Effects on sleep, mood, social interactions, activities

Interdisciplinary Progress Notes

- Effects of interventions, including possible adverse drug reactions

IDT Care Plan

- Specific interventions and follow-up plans

Seizures

SITUATION: Patient/caregiver distress and potential morbidity from uncontrolled seizure activity

Seizures are frightening and exhausting. They should be prevented if at all possible and a plan for immediate treatment should be in place for those patients who are susceptible. These include patients with a preexisting seizure disorder and those with brain tumors or brain metastases.

Causes

- Preexisting seizure disorder
- Primary cerebral neoplasm
- Metastatic disease to the brain
- Metabolic disorders
- Drug abstinence syndromes (e.g., alcohol, benzodiazapines, barbiturates, baclofen)
- New use or increased dosage of medications that lower seizure threshold in at-risk patients (e.g., phenothiazines such as proclorperazine, thorazine; butyrophenones such as haloperidol, droperidol; tricyclic antidepressants such as amitriptyline, doxepin, nortriptyline, desipramine)

Findings

- Altered mental status associated with disseminated cancer
- Headache, nausea, spontaneous projectile vomiting associated with increased intracranial pressure
- Patient may have "aura" as a prodrome to seizure activity, e.g., visual or other sensory changes such as unusual odors
- Stopping-staring behavior suggestive of "absence" type seizure activity

- Focal seizure activity
- Frank tonic-clonic activity with postictal phase

Evaluation

- Review of past medical history should reveal seizure disorder.
- Primary brain tumor or stage of nonprimary malignancy should lead to determination of seizure risk
- Differentiate muscle twitching (myoclonic jerks) and alterations in level of consciousness due to nonseizure causes
- Assess caregiver's previous experience, understanding and preparedness for seizure management
- If already on seizure prophylactic medications, review schedule, dose, and adverse effects/toxicity/drug-drug interactions
- If "breakthrough" seizure activity while on medication, may want to check blood levels or empirically alter medication regimen per physician consultation
- Determine most appropriate level of care based on patient's seizure history/risk and current care setting

Processes of Care

Psychosocial/Practical

- Educate patient/caregiver as to importance of prophylactic therapy and acute seizure management
- Protect patient from falling and from sharp or hard surfaces
- Do not actively restrain the patient or try to put anything in the mouth, but turning the patient onto a side and lifting the chin to help maintain the airway should be attempted
- Reorient patient slowly and calmly; Nothing is given to eat or drink until full recovery of sensorium and reflexes

Biomedical

- Correct readily treatable metabolic disturbances (electrolytes, glucose).
- Pharmacological management
  1. Oral prophylaxis
     a. Phenytoin
        - Loading dose: 5 mg/kg PO q3hr × 3 doses (do not use loading dose in patients with renal or hepatic failure)
        - Maintenance: 5 mg/kg PO q HS
        - Check blood levels if seizures recur (therapeutic blood levels: 10 to 20 mg/liter or 40 to 80 μmol/L)
  2. Nonoral prophylaxis (when patient unable to take oral medication)
     a. Phenobarbital 1.5 to 3 mg/kg IM qd or continuous SQ infusion of 3 to 4 mg/kg per 24 hours via a separate syringe driver (infusion system)

    b. Dexamethasone 1 mg/hr continuous SQ or IV infusion if intracranial etiology (cerebral edema, tumor) is suspected cause

    c. Midazolam 1 to 3 mg/hr continuous SQ or IV infusion

    d. Valproic acid (syrup) 250 to 500 mg tid may be given rectally via a red rubber catheter attached to small irrigation syringe

  3. Acute treatment

    a. IV access

      o Lorazapam 1 mg/min until seizures abate (up to 5 mg), or diazapam 5 to 10 mg slow IV push

      o Phenytoin IV infusion 20 mg/kg over 20 to 30 minutes in normal saline solution; An additional 5 to 10 mg/kg can be given if seizures persist.

      o If seizures do not abate with above therapies, infuse phenobarbital 20 mg/kg IV at a rate of 100 mg/min

    b. No IV access

      o Diazepam 5 to 10 mg IM, repeated q5-10min as needed to control seizure activity, followed by SQ infusion of midazolam 1 mg/hr until another prophylactic regimen can be initiated

Goals/Outcomes

- Prevention of seizures
- Preparedness of caregiver in the event of seizure activity
- Prevention of seizure-related potential morbidity/injury

Documentation in the Medical Record

Initial Assessment

- History of seizures, seizure-control regimen, and effectiveness
- Current disease process likely to pose seizure risk
- Level of understanding/preparedness of patient/caregiver regarding seizures and seizure prevention/control

Interdisciplinary Progress Notes

- Incidence and types of seizure activity
- Patient/caregiver instruction
- Understanding and adherence to seizure prevention plan
- Seizure prophylaxis toxicities/adverse effects
- Reassessment of appropriateness of level of care

IDT Care Plan

- Seizure precautions and prevention/treatment plan and interventions defined
- Follow-up and contingency plans

Skeletal Muscle and Bladder Spasms

SITUATION: Pain and associated distress from spontaneous or activity-induced muscle spasms or cramps

Causes

- Primary neuromuscular diseases
- Spinal cord or plexus injury
- Neuromuscular effects of tumor compression/infiltration
- Infection
- Bladder distention
- Metabolic disturbances (electrolyte abnormalities)
- Immobility

Findings

- "Charlie horse" of calf, thigh, low back, intercostal, neck muscles most common
- Sense of urinary urgency or crampy, colicky pain in lower pelvis; may also occur during or after voiding

Evaluation

- Elicit patient history of bladder or skeletal muscle spasms during review of systems
- Check for dysuria, urinary frequency, feeling of fullness even after voiding, inability to initiate urinary stream
- Timing of muscle spasms in relation to activity, time of day or night, position
- Consider benefits/burdens of electrolyte evaluation based on probabilities of etiology and impact of results on treatment plan

Processes of Care

- Direct primary therapy at cause if feasible and not overly burdensome

Bladder Spasms

- Pharmacological management
  1. Antibiotic therapy for infection (per culture and sensitivities, or empirical use of trimethoprim-sulfa or ciprofloxacin)
  2. Phenazopyridine 100 to 200 mg PO qid (caution about staining from pigmented urine)
  3. Lidocaine irrigation in catheterized patients: add 10 ml of 2% lidocaine to 50 ml saline irrigant, infuse and clamp catheter for 20 to 30 minutes, and then unclamp.
  4. Oxybutynin 2.5 to 5 mg PO q8-12hr prn (caution about anticholinergic effects)

- Nonpharmacological interventions
    1. Help patient reposition frequently if prone to cramps/spasms; use pillows, bolsters for support and bed rails, trapeze if patient has strength to reposition self.
    2. Passively and slowly stretch/elongate cramping muscles with continuous steady force until contraction discontinues.
    3. Gently massage with lotion.
    4. Actively warm body parts with warm moist towel.
- Pharmacological management
    1. Benzodiazepines: Titrate carefully and balance therapeutic effects against sedation and potential memory impairment.
        a. Diazepam 2 to 10 mg PO/IV titrated to effect. Repeat based on duration of response
        b. Alternatively, lorazepam 1 to 5 mg liquid concentrate can be used in patients where the oral or sublingual route is preferred
        c. Clonazepam 0.5 to 2.0 mg PO may be preferable in patients with concurrent neuropathic pain due to its purported pain relieving actions
    2. Baclofen 5 to 10 mg PO up to tid, based on response and adverse effects (sedation, urinary retention, generalized weakness)
    3. Quinine sulfate tabs (1 or 2) PO q HS as tolerated (gastrointestinal intolerance may be dose limiting)
- Intractable spasms may occasionally require special techniques (e.g., nerve blocks) to manage. Consult with a qualified and experienced expert if symptoms do not abate or treatment-related adverse effects are overly burdensome.

Goals/Outcomes

- Eliminate muscle and bladder spasms whenever possible
- Enable patient/caregiver to be able to palliate muscle spasms quickly and effectively

Documentation in the Medical Record

Initial Assessment

- Frequency, intensity, location, aggravating/inciting, alleviating characteristics and associated signs and symptoms
- Physical examination findings
- Likely etiology

Interdisciplinary Progress Notes

- Types of interventions and effects of therapies

- Instruction in prevention and treatment regimens and specific interventions
- Follow-up plan and contingencies

Skin Breakdown: Prevention and Treatment (see Table 3.6)

SITUATION: Actual or potential skin breakdown leading to patient morbidity and caregiver burden

Causes

- Pressure ulcers resulting from decreased mobility or impaired mental capacity (decubiti)
- Body fluids causing skin irritation/maceration (incontinence, ostomy sites, wound drainage, etc.)
- Itching/pruritus leading to skin excoriation
- Vascular insufficiency leading to ischemia or stasis ulcers
- Tumor erosion or infiltration
- Poor nutritional status
- Friction, abrasion from skin contact surfaces

Findings

- Reddened, irritated skin
- Sources of body fluid/wound seepage
- Nonblanching erythematous skin over pressure areas/bony prominences (e.g., sacrum, hips)
- Partial- or full-thickness ulcers, eschar formation
- Areas of skin excoriation
- Patient may or may not communicate pain.
- Putrid odor from infected wounds

Evaluation

- Elicit patient report of painful, irritating, or itchy areas.
- Physical examination of all pressure areas, especially dorsal surfaces of bedridden and immobile patients, on a daily basis
- Check for capillary filling over erythematous and blanching skin surfaces.
- Identify source(s) of bodily fluids.
- Determine cause of itching/pruritus (see Section Three - Pruritus)
- Consider superinfection of open sores/wounds/ulcers by virtue of purulence and odor.
- Assess abrasiveness of skin contact surfaces (e.g., bedclothes).

- Traditional staging of pressure ulcers (National Pressure Ulcer Advisory Panel)
  - Stage 1: Nonblanchable erythema of intact skin; the heralding lesion of skin ulceration (assessment may be difficult in darkly pigmented individuals)
  - Stage 2: Partial-thickness skin loss involving epidermis and/or dermis; The ulcer is superficial and presents clinically as an abrasion, blister, or shallow crater
  - Stage 3: Full-thickness skin loss involving damage or necrosis of subcutaneous tissue that may extend down to, but not through, underlying fascia. The ulcer presents clinically as a deep crater with or without undermining of adjacent tissue
  - Stage 4: Full-thickness skin loss with extensive destruction, tissue necrosis or damage to muscle, bone, or supporting structures (e.g., tendon or joint capsule)
- Assess and identify severity or degree of progressive/additive risk factors including:
  - General physical condition (good, fair, poor, very bad)
  - Mental condition (alert, apathetic, confused, stuporous)
  - Activity (ambulatory, walks with assistance, chairbound, bedbound)
  - Mobility (full, slightly limited, very limited, immobile)
  - Incontinence (none, occasional, frequent urinary incontinence, doubly incontinent)
  - Nutritional status (excellent, adequate, inadequate, very poor)
  - Sensory (pain) responsiveness (no impairment, slightly limited, very limited, absent)

Processes of Care

- Prevention: Caregiver education in the following areas will greatly reduce the risk of skin breakdown and the development of pressure ulcers in at risk patients (adapted from AHCPR Clinical Guideline No. 3, 1992, and No. 15, 1994).
  1. All at-risk individuals should have a systematic skin inspection at least once a day by caregiver(s) paying particular attention to the bony prominences
  2. Skin should be cleansed at the time of soiling and at routine intervals, avoiding hot water, using minimal application of friction and using mild cleansing agents that minimize irritation and dryness of the skin
  3. Use topical agents (e.g., zinc oxide preparations) that act as barriers to moisture and underpads/briefs that rapidly absorb moisture and present a quick-drying surface to the skin
  4. Avoid massage over bony prominences; Current evidence suggests that this may be harmful
  5. Minimize environmental factors leading to skin drying, such as low humidity and exposure to cold; Dry skin should be treated with moisturizers

Table 3.6. Control of Causative and Contributing Factors

Causative and Contributing Factors	Interventions
Infection	Prevention by using clean technique Treatment of infection by the use of topical and/or oral antibiotics
Excessive moisture	Prevention by keeping patient clean/dry (moisture barrier creams, diapers, pads, changing linens, etc.), especially when patient is incontinent Aggressively identify and alleviate any causes of excessive moisture
Shear and friction	Prevention by using draw sheets, not "scooting or dragging" patient across sheets, eliminating wrinkles and crumbs in linens, keep patient from sliding in bed. Treatment by quickly identifying and eliminating factors creating shear or friction
Altered nutritional status	Prevention by identifying those at risk with nutritional assessment and taking appropriate action as indicated by assessment. Encourage patient to eat/drink if this is consistent with patient goal
Unrelieved pressure	Frequent turning/repositioning, pressure relief devices such as overlay, APP mattress; **please note** that sheepskin and egg-crate mattresses are comfort measures and do not relieve pressure. Assess bony prominances frequently for signs of redness, blanching, blisters—take immediate action—do not massage area

6. Skin injury due to friction and shear forces should be minimized through proper positioning, transferring, and turning techniques. Use lubricants, protective films and dressings (e.g., hydrocolloids) and protective padding.

7. At-risk patients should be repositioned at least every 2 hours if this is consistent with established goals/preferences.

8. Apply positioning devices (e.g., pillows, foam pads) to bony prominences (e.g., knees, ankles, heels) to prevent direct contact with each other or hard surfaces.

9. Avoid positioning immobile patients with full weight on trochanter (when in lateral position)

10. Avoid uninterrupted sitting in chair/wheelchair by immobile patients if unable to shift weight from pressure points at least hourly. Balance this risk with overall patient goals/preferences.

11. Do not use donut-type devices in chairs.

Treatment

1. In order of most effective (and also most expensive) to least effective, support surfaces to prevent and treat pressure ulcers are:
   a. Air fluidized
   b. Low-air-loss
   c. Alternating-air
   d. Static flotation (air or water)
   e. Foam
   f. Standard mattress

The appropriate choice of support surface is dependent on risk factors, presence and severity of ulcers, ability of caregivers to prevent and treat ulcers, financial resources.

2. Debridement: The method of ulcer debridement chosen should be based on the patient's condition and individual goals/preferences

    a. Noninfected ulcers should be debrided with wet to dry dressings allowing autolytic debridement from enzymes normally found in wound fluids

    b. Enzymatic debridement is accomplished by applying topical debridement agents to devitalized tissue on the wound surface.

    c. The simplest form of mechanical debridement techniques include hydrotherapy and wound irrigation. Safe and effective irrigation pressures range from 4 to 15 pounds per square inch (psi); the least expensive and most effective devices that deliver pressures within this range are:

        o 60 ml piston irrigation syringe with catheter tip (4.2 psi)

        o 250 ml saline squeeze bottle with irrigation cap (4.5 psi)

        o Water Pik at lowest (#1) setting (6.0 psi)

        o 35 ml syringe with 19 gauge needle or angiocatheter (8.0 psi)

    d. Sharp debridement is rarely indicated except in those patients with a relatively long life expectancy and extensive devitalized tissue with infection; surgical consultation may be required, and pain control should be the highest priority

    e. Heel ulcers with dry eschar are an exception and need not be debrided if there is no edema, erythema, fluctuance, or drainage; Assess these wounds daily, keeping heels slightly elevated and preventing friction or pressure

3. Wound cleansing and dressings: healing and prevention of infection is more likely if fastidious wound cleansing is carried out and appropriate dressings are applied; Active cleansing needs to be balanced against inciting pain and aggravating wound trauma; Routine cleansing should be accomplished with minimal chemical or mechanical irritation/trauma

    a. Cleanse wounds with normal saline; do not use antiseptics

    b. Dress ulcers in a manner that keeps the ulcer bed moist and surrounding skin dry

    c. Wet to dry dressings should only be used for debridement

    d. There are no specific outcomes differences for different choices of moist wound dressings, so select one that is most convenient and least costly such as film and hydrocolloid dressings

    e. Only use antibiotic therapy if fastidious wound care has otherwise failed to control bacterial colonization (exudate and odor persisting after several days of routine wound care)

        o Topical antibiotic trial: silver sufadiazine or triple antibiotic, monitoring for sensitivity reactions or other adverse effects (also see "Bleeding, Oozing, and Malodorous Lesions")

- o **No** topical antiseptics, i.e., povidone-iodine, iodophor, sodium hypochlorite, hydrogen peroxide, acetic acid
- o Charcoal dressings may help reduce odor.
f. Use appropriate body substance control techniques.
g. Treat pain as indicated in "Pain."
- o Aerosolized 0.5% bupivacaine or a paste of aluminum hydroxide-magnesium hydroxide may reduce the need for, or dose of, systemic analgesics

Goals/Outcomes (see Table 3.7, a-d)

- Prevent pressure ulcers
- Eliminate adverse symptoms associated with skin breakdown if it occurs
- Minimize morbidity and added caregiver burden by adherence to skin care protocols
- Caregiver comfort with routine skin care protocols

Table 3.7a. Determining Appropriate Goals

Protocol	Patient Characteristics	Goal of Wound Care
H	Serum albumin >3.0 and/or patient eating well; <0% weight loss in past 6 months; patient ambulatory	Healing*
M	Serum albumin 2.8 to 3.0 and/or fair nutrition; ≤10% weight loss past 6 months; patient somewhat ambulatory but primarily sedentary; peripheral vascular disease and/or diabetic neuropathy	Maintenance|
C	Serum albumin <2.8; poor nutrition; >10% weight loss; primarily or totally bedbound or chairbound; peripheral vascular disease and/or diabetic neuropathy	Comfort‡

*Healing = complete healing of wound is expected.

†Maintenance = wound will not become infected or worsen, but not expected to heal.

‡Comfort = wound will not become infected, may become worse, but patient will be pain free.

Table 3.7b. Protocol H (Goal Healing)

Problem	Interventions
Wound (describe)	See earlier Treatment section.
	Assess wound for signs/symptoms of infection, treat any infection with adjunctive antibiotics.
	Manage causative and contributing factors including unrelieved pressure, shear and friction, excessive moisture, altered nutrition.
	Dietary consult as determined by nutritional assessment and IDT.
	Pain relief, if needed
	If no evidence of healing within 2 weeks after treatment initiated, reevaluate whether healing is a valid goal by assessing causative factors, nutrition, infection, vascular insufficiency. Redefine goal as indicated.
	If goal remains healing, reassess goal and discuss at IDT at least every 2 weeks.

Table 3.7c. Protocol M (Goal Maintenance)

Problem	Interventions
Wound (describe)	See earlier Treatment section.
	Dietary consult as determined by nutritional assessment and IDT
	Pain relief, if needed
	If evidence of worsening of wound, evaluate whether maintenance is a valid goal by assessing causative factors, nutrition, infection, vascular insufficiency. Redefine goal as indicated.
	If goal remains maintenance, reassess goal and discuss at IDT at least every 2 weeks.

Table 3.7d. Protocol M (Goal Maintenance)

Problem	Interventions
Wound (describe)	See earlier Treatment section.
	Pain relief, if needed
	Control odor.
	If goal remains comfort, reassess goal and discuss at IDT at least every 2 weeks.

Documentation in the Medical Record

Initial Assessment

- Findings from skin examination
- Risk factors for pressure ulcers and skin breakdown
- Needs assessment, i.e., support surfaces, caregiver capabilities

Interdisciplinary Progress Notes

- Interventions and instructions given
- Results of interventions and ongoing re-assessments

IDT Care Plan

- Specific interventions and instructions to caregiver(s)
- Follow-up plans and contingencies

Urinary Problems

SITUATION: Urinary retention or incontinence leading to patient distress or increased caregiver burden

Causes

- Benign prostatic hypertrophy in males
- Prostatic malignancy in males
- Bladder atony

- Urinary tract infection
- Medication-induced retention from anticholinergic drugs (e.g., tricyclic anti-depressants)
- Fecal impaction with secondary obstruction
- Kinked, blocked, clogged, obstructed urinary (Foley) catheter
- Patient inability to attend to toileting
- Cauda equina syndrome or other spinal/sacral plexus impairment
- Diuretic effect (especially at night)
- Stroke or other central nervous system impairment

Findings

- Patient or caregiver report of dribbling or frank incontinence
- Urinary urgency, frequency, dysuria
- Small, frequent voidings
- Infrequent voiding with "overflow" incontinence
- Bladder spasms
- Palpable bladder on physical examination
- Change in normal urine color/odor/clarity (e.g., dark, bloody, malodorous)

Evaluation

- Assess fluid intake.
- Review medications (especially diuretics, anticholinergics)
- Systems review with patient, if communicative, including abdominal pain, distention, cramps, bowel movements, change in urinary frequency, volume, color, odor, pain while voiding, etc
- Confirm or compare voiding behaviors with caregiver
- Abdominal, pelvic, perineal, genital, rectal examination as indicated by presenting symptoms/signs
- Grossly examine urine

Processes of Care

- Try to regulate fluid intake and use of diuretics to avoid nocturnal bladder filling
- Instruct patient/caregiver to have patient void in upright (sitting) position and try to initiate voiding on a fixed schedule to "train" the bladder (i.e., every 4 hours during the day)
- Adjust anticholinergic medications if at all possible, balancing relative benefits and burdens of therapies, side effects and "competing" symptom complexes
- Treat urinary tract infection and bladder spasms as per Section Three - Skeletal Muscle and Bladder Spasms
- Consider condom catheter for incontinence
- Teach caregiver care and maintenance of condom catheter system and importance of genital skin care

- Insert urinary catheter (Foley) following aseptic technique.
- Monitor initial urine output: if greater than 1000 ml, clamp catheter for 15 minutes, and then continue gravity drainage, clamping the catheter for 15 minutes for every additional 500 ml output
- Irrigate urinary catheters with sterile saline on a regular basis; discontinue if no fluid return, and consult physician
- Consult with physician if unable to pass a standard urinary catheter with minimal effort
- Instruct caregiver in care and maintenance of indwelling urinary catheter and drainage system (cleansing urinary meatus, observing for obstruction and signs of infection/inflammation around urethral opening/meatus, emptying drainage reservoir, keeping reservoir below level of the patient's bladder)
- Cranberry juice has been shown to decrease *E. coli* colony counts and may be useful in preventing or limiting inevitable bacteriuria in catheterized patients
- Lidocaine 2% ointment or 4% K-Y Jelly may help decrease pain, burning, stinging, and irritation at catheter insertion site
- Manually disempact and initiate bowel protocol per "Constipation" as needed

Goals/Outcomes

- Prevent bladder distention
- Minimize distress, additional morbidity, social isolation and caregiver burden due to incontinence

Documentation in the Medical Record

Initial Assessment

- Review of urinary symptoms, voiding patterns, fluid intake, medications
- Physical examination findings
- Effect of urinary problems on caregiver, patient self-image, and social interactions
- Effect of urinary problems on environment (odor, etc.)
- Likely cause(s) of urinary problems

Interdisciplinary Progress Notes

- Specific interventions and results
- Patient/caregiver coping

IDT Care Plan

- Etiology-specific interventions and contingencies with follow-up plan
- Plan for patient/caregiver instruction as required by circumstances

Xerostomia (Dry Mouth)

SITUATION: Dry oral mucous membranes, lips, palate, throat and tongue, often attended by cracking/bleeding oral tissues is a common finding in patients with advanced disease, causing physical and/or emotional distress to the patient and caregiver.

Causes

- Candidiasis (thrush): see "Dysphagia and Oropharyngeal Problems."
- Drugs with antisialogogic (anticholinergic) effects (e.g., tricyclic antidepressants, opioids, antihistamines, major tranquilizers)
- Radiotherapy to the head and neck region
- Dehydration
- Mouth breathing
- Hypercalcemia
- Mucositis

Findings

- Findings are generally self-evident, but the degree of distress to the patient/caregiver may need to be specifically elaborated by open-ended queries and discussion

Evaluation

- Assessment of patient and caregiver coping and concerns
- Assessment of fluid intake and interest in any type of hydration to relieve symptoms
- Physical examination of oropharynx and skin turgor

Processes of Care

- Tailor therapy to the extent of patient/caregiver concern/distress and specific cause of signs/symptoms if readily ascertained
- Symptomatic treatment can include ice chips, small sips of water, sugar-free citrus drops in patients who can control swallowing and whose airway reflexes are intact
- Lemon or lime concentrate in the imitation plastic fruit "squeezers" found in most grocery stores, is a low-cost easy-to-manage aid in symptom management for thirst/dry mouth (stimulates salivation if salivary glands are intact)
- Use of oral swabs with water is helpful, especially to assuage caregivers' concerns or perceptions of a loved one's thirst during the phase of imminent dying; similarly, application of a petrolatum-based lip balm may prevent lip cracking and be of comfort to those in attendance

- Pharmaceutical care should be directed at treatment of specific causes (e.g., candidiasis) or attempts to minimize anticholinergic drugs if possible
- Pilocarpine drops, a cholinergic drug, might stimulate salivation from remaining salivary glands in cases where radiotherapy has obliterated the majority of these tissues; The suggested dose is 5 mg PO, repeated as necessary. Excessive use might cause undesirable systemic cholinergic effects
- Salivary replacement is possible with commercially available "artificial saliva" preparations

Goals/Outcomes

- Reduction of physical distress to the patient and psychological distress to those in attendance from associated morbidity

Documentation in the Medical Record

Initial Assessment

- Patient expression of excessively dry mouth
- Physical examination findings: signs of dehydration, lip cracking, mouth breathing, oral candidiasis
- Caregiver coping
- Likely cause of symptoms/signs

Interdisciplinary Progress Notes

- Interventions and results
- Caregiver ability to carry out care and ability to cope

IDT Care Plan

- Specific interventions and follow-up plans

Appendix 1

Palliative Radiation Therapy in End-of-Life Care: Evidence-Based Utilization

Introduction

Palliative radiotherapy is an indispensable tool that can greatly enhance the quality of life in appropriately selected hospice patients with advanced cancer who still have more than a few weeks or months to live. It is primarily used to control pain due to bone metastasis. This form of therapy also can be used to prevent distressing symptoms due to tumor invasion of tissues and organs. In highly selected cases, radiotherapy can allay an "untimely" death from tumor-related hemorrhage, vascular occlusion, or respiratory distress for patients who may not yet have completed their life affairs.

Even in nonhospice environments, it is estimated that about 50% of radiation therapy treatments performed are for palliative reasons like relief of symptoms associated with primary or metastatic cancer. Yet, this important form of palliative therapy has not been used to any great extent in hospice care due to several factors, including cost, inconvenience and burden to patients, and a lack of understanding on the part of both hospice clinicians and radiation therapists about its utility in this population.

Like all interventions for palliation at the end of life, before embarking upon this form of treatment, the benefits must clearly outweigh risks and burdens. Therefore, hospice clinicians need to understand the potential role for radiation therapy (who, when, what, where and why). And radiation oncologists need to understand the contextual needs of hospice patients, their caregivers, and the system of care under which the final phase of life is being experienced.

Unfortunately, there are few radiation therapy outcome studies that can help direct the care we give to patients with advanced cancer. Much of the practice of radiation oncology is founded upon the personal experiences of therapists, as passed down by their seniors and reinforced through their own practice patterns. Additionally, widely variable approaches are taken to manage similar cases, without well-defined differences in clinical results. These factors prompt the need for critical rethinking, in order to provide a basis for rational decision-making so that hospice patients may benefit from the appropriate use of palliative radiation therapy.

Ethical Guiding Princples

(adapted and modified from Mackillop, 1996)

Palliative radiotherapy should be integrated into the comprehensive plan of care. The decision to recommend palliative radiotherapy should be based on a thorough knowledge of the patient's circumstances.

The decision to recommend palliative radiotherapy should be based upon objective information whenever possible, without adding unnecessary suffering or cost to the patient or family.

The risk-benefit analysis should include consideration of all aspects of the patient's well being. The short-term risks and benefits of palliative radiotherapy are more important than those that may or may not occur in the future.

The decision to use palliative radiotherapy should be consistent with the values and preferences of the patient.

The patient should be involved in the treatment decision to the extent that she or he wishes.

Time is precious when life is short. Delays and all waiting times should be minimized. Courses of palliative radiotherapy should be no longer than absolutely necessary to achieve the therapeutic goal. Science, not individual practice patterns or habits, should guide therapy. Palliative radiotherapy should consume no more resources than necessary.

Indications for Palliative Radiotherapy

- Pain relief
- Bone metastases
- Lung cancer causing chest pain
- Nerve root or plexus compression/invasion
  o Soft tissue infiltration
- Control of bleeding
  o Hemoptysis
  o Vaginal and rectal bleeding
- Control of fungation and ulceration
- Relief of impending or actual obstruction
  o Esophagus
  o Bronchus
  o Rectum
- Shrinkage of tumor mass(es) causing distressing symptoms
  o Brain metastasis
  o Skin lesions
- Prevention of significant functional morbidity and pain
  o Impending bone fractures (long bones, vertebral bodies)

- spinal cord compression
- Superior mediastinal obstruction (e.g., superior vena cava syndrome)

Benefits and Burdens

It takes several days to a few weeks before palliative radiation therapy creates significant therapeutic benefits. Therefore, for patients to benefit, they must have a life expectancy of at least 2 to 4 weeks. Patients whose cancer pain is not well controlled by other methods can benefit from palliative radiation therapy. Or, when analgesic therapies create dominant adverse effects, palliative radiation therapy also would be appropriate. These are examples of situations when patients *should be* considered for palliative radiation therapy.

Other times, there are cases where radiation therapy appears to be beneficial but when one views the "opportunity costs" involved, it becomes less desirable. For example, the actual time involved for a patient to receive radiation therapy treatment is short but the "opportunity cost" shows up in the transport time and associated discomfort the patient experiences. Additionally, they experience waiting time and time away from family, loved ones and the potentially meaningful activities in which they could be participating. All of these factors must be taken into account when weighing the benefits versus the costs of radiation therapy.

Many patients *can* benefit from palliative radiation therapy. Simply weigh carefully *all* of the factors when deciding on treatment.

Fractionation

Fractionation schedules (i.e., the number and timing of radiotherapy sessions and the radiation dose[s] per session) for palliative radiation therapy are not yet based upon a firm scientific footing. However, there is much evidence (supported in the following paragraphs) that suggests shorter courses of treatment are just as effective as more protracted schedules. An additional benefit of short courses is they incur less acute toxicity in the patient. With fewer trips to a treatment facility, patients also experience less discomfort and have more time to spend in other endeavors. Additionally, palliative radiation therapy can be costly in comparison to the likelihood of the improved outcomes it may offer.

Bone Pain

Where palliative radiation therapy is indicated, there is much evidence to suggest, under most circumstances, that a short course (one to five doses) is as effective as more protracted treatment schedules (10–20 fractions) and incurs less acute toxicity. The most recent clinical trials have strongly suggested that single fraction therapy is very effective for the treatment of metastatic bone pain.

Non–Small Cell Lung Cancer

The Medical Research Council trials in Great Britain compared a regimen of 17 Gy in two fractions with 30 Gy in two fractions and a single 10-Gy fraction to the two-fraction treatment in patients with poor performance status (i.e., hospice eligible). The short course therapy (one or two fractions) proved to be as effective as the longer course approach without incurring any greater toxicity.

Brain Metastases

The data for treating cerebral metastases are similar to that for bone disease. The Radiation Therapy Oncology Group clinical trials and European studies suggest that a 3-day course of treatment is as effective as a more protracted regimen.

Fractionation Conclusions

Based upon historical and mounting contemporary evidence, one, two, or a few (at the most) fractions represent the most beneficial approach to palliative radiation therapy, when indicated in patients with limited life expectancy. It would be against the interests of any patient to propose, no less institute, a protracted fractionation schedule that is time consuming, creates patient discomfort and is costly in comparison to evidence of the likelihood of improved outcomes compared with a brief intervention.

The approach toward minimal palliative radiotherapy has not yet become the norm in the United States, although it needs to be invoked as a standard of care for hospice patients unless new data emerge to the contrary. Disagreement with such an approach should be challenged on the basis of the scientific evidence, and professionalism in all such discussions should prevail, with a focus on what serves the best interests of the patient.

Acute Toxicity

There are several potential adverse effects associated with radiation therapy. Most develop a week or two after treatment when tumor cell death is at its peak. These after effects can be anticipated and should be prevented or treated in order to minimize symptoms.

Fatigue

Frequently, patients voice symptoms of fatigue. The cause of treatment-related fatigue during the actual course of therapy is not well understood. It may be an effect of radiation treatment, per se, or the exertion required for the patient to attend such therapy.

A brief course of psychostimulants may be a creative and relatively benign means to treat fatigue. As of yet, use of low-dose psychostimulants, e.g., methylphenidate, has not yet been formally studied for this indication.

Skin Symptoms

The most common finding is localized erythema, which resolves in 2 to 3 weeks after completion of therapy. If there is any discomfort associated with it, unbroken skin can be treated with a topical steroid cream (e.g., 1% hydrocortisone). If skin breakdown occurs, this should be treated like any open sore or ulcer (e.g., decubitus care) in order to prevent secondary infection.

Visceral Symptoms

There is a risk of nausea and vomiting during the course of treatment, and these symptoms may persist for a few days following the completion of radiation therapy.

Antiemetic therapy should adhere to usual processes of care, starting with first-line approaches (see section III.18) and progressing to dexamethasone and then ondansetron or granisetron for intractable cases, as necessary.

Diarrhea may occur shortly after exposure of the intestines to radiation therapy. Anticipation of this occurrence by switching to a low-fiber diet (for patients who are eating a full range of foods) may prevent it. If diarrhea does occur, follow established simple processes of care, prescribing loperamide or diphenoxylate as initial therapies.

Dysuria, Urinary Frequency

These symptoms can occur after brief exposure of the bladder to ionizing radiation. Treatment with phenazopyridine and a low dose of an anticholinergic agent (e.g., amitriptyline 10 mg HS) may provide symptomatic relief.

Conclusion

The sum of the current scientific evidence suggests that palliative radiotherapy is underutilized in end-of-life care. When it is proffered, the frequency of treatment regimens commonly exceeds the likely benefits to be derived, adding greater burden than benefit. An evidence-based understanding and application of its role in symptom management by all healthcare providers and caregivers at this crucial time in patients' lives will lead to an improvement in end of life care. As with most therapeutic options, appropriate patient selection and informed consent are the foundation of good care. It is now up to hospice professionals and radiation oncologists to act in accordance with the evidence at hand.

Bibliography

Anonymous. Inoperable non-small-cell lung cancer (NSCLC): a medical research council randomised trial of palliative radiotherapy with two fractions or ten fractions. Report to the Medical Research Council by its Lung Cancer Working Party. *Br J Cancer* 1991;63:265–270.

Anonymous. A Medical Research Council (MRC) randomised trial of palliative radiotherapy with two fractions or a single fraction in patients with inoperable non-small-cell lung cancer (NSCLC) and poor performance status. Medical Research Council Lung Cancer Working Party. *Br J Cancer* 1992;65:934–941.

Allen KL, Johnson TW, Hibbs GG. Effective bone palliation as related to various treatment regimes. *Cancer* 1976;37:984–987.

Arcangeli G, Micheli A, Giannarelli D, et al. The responsiveness of bone metastases to radiotherapy: The effect of site, histology and radiation dose on pain relief. *Radiother Oncol* 1989;14:95–101.

Barak F, Werner A, Walach N, Horn Y. The palliative efficacy of a single dose of radiation in treatment of symptomatic osseous metastases. *Int J Radiat Oncol Biol Phys* 1987;13:1233–1235.

Bates T. A review of local radiotherapy in the treatment of bone metastases and cord compression. *Int J Radiat Oncol Biol Phys* 1992;23:217–221.

Blitzer PH. Reanalysis of the RTOG study of the palliation of syptomatic osseous metastasis. *Cancer* 1985;55:468–1472.

Borgelt B, Gelber R, Kramer S, et al. The palliation of brain metastases: Final results of the first two studies by the radiation therapy oncology group. *Int J Radiat Oncol Biol Phys* 1980;6:1–9.

Burmeister BH, Probert JC. Half body irradiation for the palliation of bone metastases. *Australas Radiol* 1990;34:317–319.

Cheng DS, Seitz CB, Eyre HJ. Nonoperative management of femoral, humeral, and acetabular metastases in patients with breast carcinoma. *Cancer* 1980;45:1533–1537.

Chow E, Harris K, Fan G, Tsao M, Sze WM. Palliative radiotherapy trials for bone metastases: A systematic review. *J Clin Oncol* 2007;25(11):1423–1436.

Coia LR, Hanks GE, Martz K. Practice patterns of palliative care for the United States 1984–1985. *Int J Radiat Oncol Biol Phys* 1988;14:1261–1269.

Coia LR, Owen JB, Maher EJ, et al. Factors affecting treatment patterns of radiation oncologists in the United States in the palliative treatment of cancer. *Clin Oncol* 1992;4:6–10.

Cole DJ. A randomized trial of single treatment versus conventional fractionation in the palliative radiotherapy of painful bone metastases. *Clin Oncol* 1989;1:59–62.

Crellin AM, Marks A, Maher EJ. Why don't British radiotherapists give single fractions of radiotherapy for bone metastases? *Clin Oncol* 1989;1:63–66.

Dawson R, Currow D, Stevens G, Morgan G, Barton MB. Radiotherapy for bone metastases: A critical appraisal of outcome measures. *J Pain Symptom Manage* 1999;17:208–218.

Dodwell D, Bond M, Elwell C, et al. Effect of medical audit on prescription of palliative radiotherapy. *Br Med J* 1993;307:24–25.

Duncan G, Duncan EW, Maher EJ. Patterns of palliative radiotherapy in Canada. *Clin Oncol* 1993;5:92–97.

Garmatis CJ, Chu FCH. The effectiveness of radiation therapy in the treatment of bone metastases from breast cancer. *Radiology* 1978;126:235–237.

Gaze MN, Kelly CG, Kerr GR, et al. Pain relief and quality of life following radiotherapy for bone metastases: A randomised trial of two fractionation schedules. *Radiother Oncol* 1997;45:109–116.

Gilbert HA, Kagan AR, Nussbaum H, et al. Evaluation of radiation therapy for bone metastases: Pain relief and quality of life. *AJR Am J Roentgenol* 1977;129:1095–1096.

Haie MC, Pellae CB, Laplanche A, et al. Results of a randomized clinical trial comparing two radiation schedules in the palliative treatment of brain metastases. *Radiother Oncol* 1993;26:111–116.

Hartsell WF, Scott CB, Bruner DW, Scarantino CW, Ivker RA, Roach M 3rd, Suh JH, Demas WF, Movsas B, Petersen IA, Konski AA, Cleeland CS, Janjan NA, DeSilvio M. Randomized trial of short- versus long-course radiotherapy for palliation of painful bone metastases. *J Natl Cancer Inst* 2005;97(11):798–804.

Hoskin PJ, Ford HT, Harmer CL. Hemibody irradiation for metastatic bone pain in two histologically distinct groups of patients. *Clin Oncol* 1989;1:67–69.

Hoskin PJ, Price P, Easton D, et al. A prospective randomised trial of 4 Gy and 8 Gy single doses in the treatment of metastatic bone pain. *Radiother Oncol* 1992;23:74–78.

Janjan NA. An emerging respect for palliative care in radiation oncology. *J Palliat Med* 1998;1:83–88.

Jensen NH, Roesdahl K. Single dose irradiation of bone metastases. *Acta Radiol* 1976;15:337–339.

Kirkbride P, Barton R. Palliative radiation therapy. *J Palliat Med* 1999;2:87–97.

Kuban DA, DelbrIDTe T, el Mahdu AM, et al. Half body irradiation for treatment of widely metastatic carcinoma of the prostate. *J Urol* 1989;141:572–574.

Lawton PA, Maher EJ. Treatment strategies for advanced and metastatic cancer in Europe. *Radiother Oncol* 1991;22:1–6.

Mackillop WJ. The principles of palliative radiotherapy: A radiation oncologist's perspective. *Can J Oncol* 1996(suppl):5–11.

Mackillop WJ, Quirt CF. Measuring the accuracy of prognostic judgements in oncology. *J Clin Epidemiol* 1997;50:21–29.

Madsen EL. Painful bone metastasis: Efficacy of radiotherapy assessed by the patients. *Int J Radiat Oncol Biol Phys* 1983;9:1775–1779.

Maher EJ, Coia L, Duncan G, Lawton PA. Treatment strategies in advanced and metastatic cancer: Differences in attitude between the USA, Canada and Europe. *Int J Radiat Oncol Phys* 1992;23:239–244.

Maher EJ, Timothy A, Squire CF. Audit: The use of radiotherapy for NSCLC in the UK. *Clin Oncol* 1993;5:72–79.

Martin WMC. Multiple daily fractions of radiation in the palliation of pain from bone metastases. *Clin Radiol* 1983;34:245–249.

McCloskey SA, Tao ML, Rose CM, Fink A, Amadeo AM. National survey of perspectives of palliative radiation therapy: Role, barriers, and needs. *Cancer J* 2007;13(2):130–137.

McQuay HJ, Carroll D, Moore RA. Radiotherapy for painful bone metastases. *Clin Oncol* 1997;9:150–154.

Mithal NP, Needham PR, Hoskin PJ. Retreatment with radiotherapy for painful bone metastases. *Int J Radiat Oncol Biol Phys* 1994;29:1011–1014.

Munro A, Sebag-Montefiore D. Opportunity cost—A neglected aspect of cancer treatment. *Br J Cancer* 1992;65:309–310.

Nag S, Shah V. Once a week lower hemibody irradiation for metastatic cancers. *Int J Radiat Oncol Biol Phys* 1986;12:1003–1005.

Needham PR, Hoskin PJ. Radiotherapy for painful bone metastases. *Palliat Med* 1994; 8:95–104.

Nielsen OS, Bentzen SM, Sandberg E, et al. Randomized trial of single dose versus fractionated palliative radiotherapy of bone metastases. *Radiother Oncol* 1998; 47:233–240.

Nielsen P, Munroe A, Tannock I. Management policy for treatment of bone metastases. *J Clin Oncol* 1991;9:509–524

Niewald M, Tkocz HJ, Abel U, et al. Rapid course radiation therapy vs. more standard treatment: A randomized trial for bone metastases. *Int J Radiat Oncol Biol Phys* 1996;36:1085–1089.

Okawa T, Kita M, Goto M, et al. Randomized prospectie clinical study of small, large and twice a day fractionation radiotherapy for painful metastases. *Radiother Oncol* 1988;13:99–104.

Penn CRH. Single dose and fractionated irradiation for osseous metastases. *Clin Radiol* 1976;27:405–408.

Poulter CA, Cosmatos D, Rubin P, et al. A report of RTOG 8206: A phase III study of whether the addition of single dose hemibody irradiation is more effective than local field irradiation alone in the treatment of symptomatic osseous metastases. *Int J Radiat Oncol Biol Phys* 1992;23:207–214.

Priestman TJ, Bullimore JA, Godden TP, et al. The Royal College of Radiologists' fractionation survey. *Clin Oncol* 1989;1:39–46.

Price P, Hoskin PJ, Easton D, et al. Low dose single fraction radiotherapy in the treatment of metastatic bone pain: A pilot study. *Radiother Oncol* 1988;12:297–300.

Richter MP, Coia LR. Palliative radiation therapy. *Sein Oncol* 1985;12:375–383.

Stevens G, Firth I. Patterns of fractionation for palliation of bone metastases. *Australas Radiol* 1995;39:31–35.

Salazar OM, Rubin P, Hendrickson FR, et al. Single dose half body irradiation for palliation of multiple bone metastases from solid tumors. Final Radiation Therapy Oncology Group Report. *Cancer* 1986;58:29–36.

Schocker JD, Brady LW. Radiation therapy for bone metastasis. *Clin Orthop Rel Res* 1982;169:38–43.

Tong D, Gillick L, Hendrickson FR. The palliation of symptomatic osseous metastases. Final results of the RTOG study. *Cancer* 1982;50:893–899.

Vargha ZI, Arvin SG, Boland J. Single dose radiation therapy in the palliation of metastatic disease. *Radiology* 1969;93:1181–1184.

Wai MS, Mike S, Ines H, Malcolm M. Palliation of metastatic bone pain: Single fraction versus multifraction radiotherapy—A systematic review of the randomised trials. *Cochrane Database Syst Rev* 2004;(2):CD004721.

Wilkins MF, Keen CW. Hemi body radiotherapy in the management of metastatic carcinoma. *Clin Radiol* 1987;38:267–268.

Yarnold JR. Bone Pain Trial: A prospective randomized trial comparing single dose of 8 Gy and a multifraction radiotherapy schedule in the treatment of metastatic bone pain. *Br J Cancer* 1988;78:6.

Zelefsky MJ, Scher HI, Forman JD, et al. Palliative hemiskeletal irradiation for widespread metastatic prostate cancer: A comparison of single dose and fractionated regimens. *Int J Radiat Oncol Biol Phys* 1989;17:1281–1285.

Appendix 2

Principles of Pharmacotherapy

General Principles

- Maximize efficacy (therapeutic effect)
- Minimize adverse effects (toxicity)
- Minimize cost (conscious and conscientious resource utilization)

In most cases this means
- Use generic formulations when this option exists
- Only use more costly formulations when there is a specific indication
- Convenience alone (not to be confused with significant issues of compliance) or personal preferences of the prescriber are rarely, if ever, sufficient reasons for medication selection

Application of general principles to opioid prescribing practices
- Use the oral or transdermal route unless there are contraindications
- Contraindications to oral administration: patient is NPO, short bowel syndrome, malabsorption syndrome, dumping syndrome, intractable nausea and vomiting
- Contraindications to transdermal administration: fever, diaphoresis, excessive skin sensitivity, extremes of cachexia or obesity
- Consider the rectal route when oral/transdermal routes are contraindicated, but this is an area where personal issues (patient and caregiver) need to be respected
- Use continuous/sustained release formulations for continuous (unremitting) pain
- Use immediate-release, short-acting formulations for breakthrough pain or for rescue analgesia (more than 3 or 4 doses per day should trigger consideration of upward titration of the long-acting formulation)
- Breakthrough pain doses should be from 10% to 20% of the 24-hour dose of total analgesic (e.g., if a patient is taking 60 mg continuous release morphine by mouth every 12 hours, the breakthrough pain dose should be about 18 mg [range of 12 to 24 mg] morphine or its equivalent)
- Only use alternative or more costly formulations if there is a specific contraindication to a lower cost formulation

- If a patient's pain is well controlled on an analgesic regimen at the time of admission, take a thorough medication history, including past reactions/experiences with other opioid analgesics, and only change medications if specific drug-related problems develop
- Use U.S. Food and Drug Administration (FDA)-approved pharmaceuticals and routes of administration (predictable and proven uptake and absorption) unless there is a clinical need for which there is no approved product available. Under these circumstances, compounding is justified

CRITICAL THINKING AND APPLICATION OF SOUND PRINCIPLES OF PRESCRIBING NEED TO BE THE FIRST STEPS OF EVERY MEDICATION ORDER

Drug Interactions

Likelihood of drug interactions occurring with commonly used drugs

Drug Class	Frequent	Occasional	Uncommon
OPIOIDS			
Codeine		*	
Fentanyl			*
Hydromorphone			*
Methadone		*	
Morphine			*
Oxycodone	*		
NEUROLEPTICS			
Haloperidol	*		
Chlorpromazine		*	
ANTIDEPRESSANTS			
Tricyclics	*		
SSRIs	*		
MAO inhibitors	*		
ANTIEMETICS			
Metoclopramide			*
Ondansetron			*
CORTICOSTEROIDS	*		
BENZODIAZAPINES		*	

Bibliography

Caraco J, Sheller J, Wood AJJ. Pharmacogenetic determination of the effects of codeine and prediction of drug interactions. *J Pharmacol Exp Ther* 1996;278:1165–1174.

Cowen P. Antidepressant drugs. In: Aronson J (ed), *Side Effects of Drugs Annual* 1997; 20: 6–10.

Crewe HK, Lennard MS, Tucker GT, et al. The effect of selective serotonin re-uptake inhibitors on cytochrome P450 (CYP 2D6) activity in human liver microsomes. *Br J Clin Pharm* 1992;34:262–265.

Fine PG. *Diagnosis and Treatment of Breakthrough Pain.* Oxford University Press, New York, 2008.

Fine PG, Portenoy RK. *Clinical Guide to Opioid Analgesia,* 2nd Edition. Vendome Press, New York, 2007.

Gear R, Miaskowski C, Heller PH, et al. Benzodiazapine mediated antagonism of opioid analgesia. *Pain* 1997;71:25–29.

Kivisto K, Kroemer HK, Eichelbaum M. The role of human cytochrome P450 enzymes in the metabolism of anticancer agents: Implications for drug interactions. *Br J Clin Pharm* 1995;40:523–530.

Rizack M, Gardner D. The Medical Letter—Drug Interaction Program 1998;10.

Appendix 3

Ketamine Protocol

Background to Ketamine

Ketamine is a dissociative anaesthetic agent that has analgesic properties in sub-anaesthetic doses. Ketamine is the most potent NMDA receptor channel blocker available for clinical use. Ketamine has other actions that may also contribute to its analgesic effect, including interactions with other calcium and sodium channels, cholinergic transmission, noradrenergic and serotoninergic re-uptake inhibition, and μ, δ, and κ opioid–like effects. Ketamine also appears to have an antidepressant effect in patients with major depression. Generally, ketamine is used in addition to morphine or alternative strong opioid when further opioid increments have been ineffective or precluded by unacceptable undesirable effects. When used in this way, ketamine is generally administered PO or SC. It can also be administered IM, IV, SL, intranasally, PR, and spinally (preservative-free formulation).

Indications

- Refractory cancer pain, under following circumstances
  o "Maximal" titration of opioid (to include trial of oral methadone) with prior opioid rotation
  o Where side effects of opiates have become a limiting factor in further titration despite opiate rotation
  o Where oral route for other neuropathic agents not possible
  o Evidence of opioid-related hyperalgesia
  o Opioid tolerance suspected on basis of rapid escalation of opioid dose without evidence of progressive or new disease
- Ischemic, inflammatory, myofascial pain or severe neuropathic pain where unresponsive/limited response to standard therapies

Contraindications

- Raised intracranial pressure, epilepsy

Cautions

- Hypertension, cardiac failure, history of cerebrovascular accidents
- Plasma concentration increased by **diazepam**

Relative Treatment Exclusions

- Recent psychiatric hospitalization, suicide attempt or ECT in last month
- History of psychosis/schizophrenia
- History of recent seizures
- **Uncontrolled** raised intracranial pressure due to brain metastases or hydrocephalus
- Severe labile hypertension or poorly controlled cardiac arrhythmia
- COPD with associated hypercarbia

Potential General Side Effects

- Although 40% of patients receiving anesthetic doses via IV/SC route have some side effect, there is a very low incidence of adverse effects reported with subanesthetic doses of ketamine used for pain control. Potential adverse effects include increased oral secretions, hypertension, tachycardia; psychotomimetic phenomena (euphoria, dsyphoria, blunted affect, psychomotor retardation, vivid dreams, nightmares, poor concentration, illusions, hallucinations, altered body image), delirium, dizziness, diplopia, blurred vision, nystagmus, altered hearing, and erythema and pain at injection site.
- Psychotomimetic side effects generally can be controlled by **diazepam, midazolam,** or **haloperidol/chlorpromazine.**

Guidelines for Use (SC/IV or Oral)

- Initiation only by approval of experienced physician
- Administration/dose escalation by experienced physician only
- Nurse in charge and assigned to patient has received in-service on ketamine*
- Indications for use met
- Accurate weight for patient
- Determine patients prognosis
  o If short (days to weeks), use continuous infusion

o If longer (weeks to months), consider "burst" ketamine (reduces tachy-phylaxis/tolerance issues); oral ketamine (see below).

Required monitoring

- Monitoring required during initial induction period and then every 6 hours
  o Vital signs: Pulse, blood pressure, pulse oximetry
  o Elicit and record pain score
  o Psychomimetic effects
  o Monitor respiratory secretions
  o Headaches

Continuous IV/SC Infusion Protocol

Equipment
- Small syringes
- Saline boluses
- Ketamine
- Infusion pump available

Adjuvant Medications Available at Bedside
- Diazepam 5 to 10 mg (seizures unlikely at these doses)
- Chlorpromazine 12.5 to 25 mg every 6 hours: psychomimetic effects
- Glycopyrrolate 0.2 to 0.4 mg IV/SC for secretions
- Labetalol 2.5 mg every 6 hours IV for hypertension/tachycardia

Continuous Infusion Protocol	Time	Pain score	BP	Pulse	Other	Medications given
Give 0.1mg/kg IV/SC bolus of e.g. 70kg ketamine: *patient = 7 mg bolus*	00.00					
Reduce opiate infusion by 50%						
Wait 15 minutes then , monitor-	00.15					
If good response consider this dose for basis of infusion: if partial or minimal response give 2nd bolus at double dose: *e.g., 0.2 mg/kg*						
Observe for response over 15 minutes	00.30					
If partial response: Give 3rd bolus maximal dose: up to 0.5 mg/kg but suggest max *20–30 mg bolus*	00.30					
Monitor q15min and observe duration of effective response(usually 15–30 minutes, occasionally hours)	00.45					

Calculate mg/hr rate from duration of
   response: *e.g., if 10 mg lasts 20 minutes,*
   then infusion rate is 30 mg/hr

Give additional bolus (at last bolus rate)   00.50
   and then start infusion.

Infusion concentration 1 to 5 mg/ml,
   e.g., If 1 mg/1 ml concentration, run
   at 30 ml/hr.

May be able to discontinue opiate
   infusion but have PCA/bolus opiate
   available q10–15min

Reassess in 24 hours   24.50

Good control—no change

Titration required—increase infusion rate by 0.05 to 0.1 mg/kg per hour

Continue to monitor for undesirable psychotomimetic effects, excessive salivation,
   tachycardia

"Burst" Ketamine Protocol SC/IV

Method "A" (SC):

Initial dose: 100 mg given over 24 hours

Increase after 24 hours to 300 mg/24 hr if 100 mg ineffective

Increase then to 500 mg/24 hr if 300 mg not effective

Stop 3 days after last dose increment

Method "B" (IV):

Single 4-hour IV infusion of 0.6 mg/kg

Oral Protocol

Use direct from vial or dilute to 50 mg/5 ml using flavoring such as Kool-Aid to mask
bitterness (i.e., add 10 ml vial of ketamine 100 mg/ml injectable to 90 ml purified water, store
in refridgerator up to 1 week):

Initial dose 10–25 mg tid-qid and prn

Titrate to optimal effect in dose increments of 10 mg to maximum dose 50 mg qid

Onset of action: 30 minutes; half-life 3 hours ketamine and 12 hours norketamine

Maximum reported dose is 200 mg po qid

If hallucinations, mood disturbance, nightmares, or drowsiness occurs, give smaller doses
more frequently. Drowsiness may also improve with reducing opiate by 25% to 50%.

Pharmacy Notes

- Ketamine is miscible with dexamethasone, haloperidol, metocloperamide,
  midazolam, and morphine.
- Ketamine can be irritant; dilute in largest volume feasible of 0.9% normal saline
- Usual dose concentration: 1 to 5 mg/ml
- Inflammation at infusion site can be helped by 1% hydrocortisone cream or
  by adding dexamethasone 0.5 to 1 mg to the infusion (dilute in 5 to 10 ml
  normal saline and then add to ketamine).

Bibliography

Fine PG. Ketamine: From anesthesia to palliative care. *AAHPM Bull* 2003;3(3):1–6.

Fine PG. Low-dose ketamine in the management of opioid resistant terminal cancer pain. *J Pain Symptom Manage* 1999;17:296–300.

Jackson K, Ashby M, Martin P, et al: 'Burst' ketamine for refractory cancer pain: An open-label audit of 39 patients. *J Pain Symptom Manage* 2001;22:834–842.

Meller S: Ketamine: Relief from chronic pain through actions at the NMDA receptor? *Pain* 1996;69:435–436.

Mitchell A: Does ketamine improve ischemic limb pain? Results from a double blind randomized control trial. Poster Abstract, Pain Society Annual Scientific Meeting, 27–30 March 2001, Poster 42: 50.

Slatkin NE, Rhiner M: Ketamine in the treatment of refractory cancer pain: Case report, rationale and methodology. *Supportive Oncol* 2003;1(4):287–293.

www.palliativedrugs.com/book.php?ketamine.

Appendix 4

Clinical/Functional Assessment

New York Heart Association Classification—A Clinical Guide

Stage I heart disease: No symptoms of heart disease [PPS 100]
Stage II heart disease: Symptoms of heart disease at MORE than normal activity [PPS 80]
Stage III heart disease: Symptoms of heart disease at LESS than normal activity [PPS 60]
Stage IV heart disease: Symptoms of heart disease at REST or at MINIMAL activity [PPS ≤50]

Functional Assesment Staging (FAST)

The Functional Assessment Staging Tool is a useful means of codifying far advanced dementing illness, and it has some prognostic value as a component to hospice eligibility determination under the current provisions of the Medicare Hospice Benefit. This was first published by Reisburg [Reisburg B. Functional assessment staging (FAST). Psychopharmacol Bull 1988;24:653–659] and can be located at: http://www.acsu.buffalo.edu/~drstall/fast.html.

Appendix 5

Palliative Performance Scale (PPS)

%	Ambulation	Activity and Evidence of Disease	Self-Care	Intake	Level of Consciousness
100	Full	Normal activity, no evidence of disease	Full	Normal	Full
90	Full	Normal activity, some evidence of disease	Full	Normal	Full
80	Full	Normal activity with effort, some evidence of disease	Full	Normal or reduced	Full
70	Reduced	Unable to do normal work, some evidence of disease	Full	Normal or reduced	Full
60	Reduced	Unable to do hobby or housework, significant disease	Occasional assistance necessary	Normal or reduced	Full or confusion
50	Mainly sit/lie	Unable to do any work, extensive disease	Considerable assistance required	Normal or reduced	Full or confusion
40	Mainly in bed	As above	Mainly assistance	Normal or reduced	Full, drowsy, or confusion
30	Totally bed bound	As above	Total care	Reduced	Full, drowsy, or confusion
20	As above	As above	Total care	Minimal sips	Full, drowsy, or confusion
10	As above	As above	Total care	Mouth care only	Drowsy or coma
0	Death	—	—	—	—

Adapted with permission from Anderson G, Downing M, Hill J, Casorso L, Lerch N. Palliative Performance Scale (PPS): A new tool. *J Palliat Care* 1996;12(1):5–11.

Index

AA (Alcoholics Anonymous),
    31
abuse in homes
    assessments, 19–20
    documentation and medical
        records, 21
    processes of care, 20
accreditation entities,
    documentation, 16
advance care planning/health
    care intervention directives
    assessments, 21
    documentation in medical
        record, 23
    findings, 21
    goals and outcomes, 23
    processes of care, 22
aesthenia (weakness). See
    fatigue, weakness
    (aesthenia), excessive
    sedation
agitation and anxiety
    assessment, 56
    causes, 56
    documentation in medical
        record, 60
    evaluation, 57–58
    findings, 56–57
    goals/outcomes, 60
    IDT care plan, 60
    pharmacotherapy, 58–59
    processes of care, 58–60
air hunger (dyspnea)
    assessment, 52
    causes, 51
    documentation in medical
        record, 55–56
    findings, 51
    goals/outcomes, 55
    IDT care plan, 55
    pharmacotherapy, 53
    processes of care, 52–55
AL-ANON (12 Step Program),
    31
anorectal problems. See
    diarrhea and anorectal
    problems
anorexia and cachexia
    assessment, 63
    documentation in medical
        record, 63
    evaluation, 61
    findings, 61

goals/outcomes, 63
IDT care plan, 63
pharmacotherapy, 62
processes of care, 62–63
ascites. See edema (peripheral
    edema, ascites,
    lymphedema)
assessments
    abuse in home, 19–20
    advance care planning and
        directives, 21
    completion of worldly
        business/life closure, 28
    cultural differences, 33
    denial, 34
    domains
        diagnostic studies, 5
        history, 4
        physical examination, 4
    grief reactions, 36
    living environment, finances,
        support systems, 40
    suicide, risk/prevention/
        coping with, 45
assessments
    (clinical/functional)
    functional assessment
        staging (FAST), 161
    NY Heart Association
        Classification/Clinical
        Guide, 161
assessments (clinical pro-
    cesses/symptom
    management)
    agitation/anxiety, 56
    air hunger (dyspnea), 52
    anorexia and cachexia,
        63
    belching/burping
        (eructation), 65
    confusion/delirium, 73
    constipation, 74, 76
    coughing, 78
    depression, 82
    diarrhea and anorectal
        problems, 85
    dysphagia/oropharyngeal
        problems, 87
    edema, 90
    fatigue, weakness, excessive
        sedation, 93
    fever and diaphoresis, 95
    hiccups, 97

    imminent death, 100
    insomnia/nocturnal
        restlessness, 104
    malodorous lesions, 70
    nausea/vomiting, 108
    pain, 127
    pruritus, 130
    seizures, 132
    skin breakdown, 140
    spasms, skeletal
        muscle/bladder, 134
    urinary problems, 142
    xerostomia (dry mouth),
        143
assisted death, 12

bathroom safety, 41
bed safety, 42
belching and burping
    (eructation)
    assessments, 65
    causes, 63–64
    documentation in medical
        record, 65
    goals/outcomes, 65
    IDT care plan, 65
    pharmacotherapy, 65
    processes of care, 65
benefits and burdens
    assessment of, for hospice
        care, 7f
    balancing of, for all
        interventions, 6–7
    define/evaluation for
        therapeutic
        interventions, 3
    palliative radiation therapy,
        147
bladder spasms. See spasms,
    skeletal muscle/bladder
bleeding, oozing, malodorous
    lesions
    causes, 66
    documentation in medical
        record, 70
    evaluation, 67
    findings, 66–67
    goals/outcomes, 69–70
    process of care, 68–69
body image, changes/loss of
    independence
    assessment, 24
    findings, 23–24

body image (*continued*)
  goals/outcomes, 25
  processes of care, 24–25
burdens
  of all interventions,
    balancing, 6–7
  anticipation attempts, 3
  assessment of, 7*f*

cachexia. *See* anorexia and
    cachexia
care conference format, for
    IDTs, 9–10
care plans. *See*
    interdisciplinary teams
    (IDTs), care plans
case managers, needs
    assessment
  after death, 14
  few months before death, 12
  last few days/weeks, 13–14
  6 months or longer before
    death, 11
causes
  agitation and anxiety, 56
  air hunger (dyspnea), 51
  belching and burping
    (eructation), 63–64
  bleeding, oozing,
    malodorous lesions, 66
  confusion/delirium, 70–71
  constipation, 74
  coughing, 77
  depression, 79
  diarrhea/anorectal
    problems, 82
  domains of, 4
  dysphagia/oropharyngeal
    problems, 85
  edema (ascites,
    lymphedema), 88
  fatigue, weakness, excessive
    sedation, 91
  fever and diaphoresis, 93
  hiccups, 95
  insomnia/nocturnal
    restlessness, 101
  nausea and vomiting, 105
  pain, 109
  pruritus, 128
  seizures, 130
  skin breakdown
    (prevention/treatment),
    135
  spasms, skeletal
    muscle/bladder, 133
  urinary problems, 140–141
  xerostomia (dry mouth),
    143
certified nurse assistant
    (CNA). *See* CNA/HHA
chaplain, needs assessment
  after death, 15

few months before death,
    13
  last few days/weeks, 14
  6 months or longer before
    death, 12
children
  grief reactions in, 38*t*–39*t*
  medical supply protection
    from, 42, 43
clinical/functional assessment
  functional assessment
    staging (FAST), 161
  NY Heart Association
    Classification/Clinical
    Guide, 161
clinical processes/symptom
    management
  agitation and anxiety, 56–60
  air hunger (dyspnea), 50–56
  anorexia and cachexia,
    61–63
  belching/burping
    (eructation), 63–65
  bleeding, oozing,
    malodorous lesions,
    66–70
  confusion/delirium, 70–74
  constipation, 74–76
  coughing, 77–78
  death, imminent, 97–100
  depression, 79–82
  diarrhea/anorectal
    problems, 82–85
  dysphagia/oropharyngeal
    problems, 85–88
  edema (peripheral, ascites,
    lymphedema), 88–90
  fatigue, weakness, excess
    sedation, 91–93
  fever/diaphoresis, 93–95
  hiccups, 95–97
  insomnia/nocturnal
    restlessness, 101–104
  nausea/vomiting, 105–108
  pain, 108–127
  pruritus, 128–130
  seizures, 130–132
  skin breakdown, 135–140
  spasms, skeletal
    muscle/bladder, 133–135
  urinary problems, 140–142
  xerostomia, 143–144
closure of worldly
    business/life. *See* worldly
    business/life closure,
    completion of
CNA/HHA, needs assessment
  after death, 14
  few months before death,
    12
  last few days/weeks, 14
  6 months or longer before
    death, 11

confusion/delirium
  assessments, 73
  causes, 70–71
  documentation in medical
    record, 73–74
  evaluation, 71–72
  findings, 71
  goals/outcomes, 73
  IDT care plan, 74
  pharmacotherapy, 72
  processes of care, 72–73
constipation
  assessments, 74, 76
  causes, 74
  documentation in medical
    record, 76
  evaluation, 74–75
  findings, 74
  goals/outcomes, 76
  IDT care plan, 76
  pharmacotherapy, 75–76
  processes of care, 75–76
controlled substances,
    misuse/abuse
  assessment, 31
  documentation in medical
    record, 32
  findings, 30
  goals/outcomes, 32
  processes of care, 31–32
coughing
  assessments, 78
  causes, 77
  documentation in medical
    record, 78
  evaluation, 77
  findings, 77
  goals/outcomes, 78
  IDT care plan, 78
  processes of care, 78
counselors, grief support, 14,
    15, 29
cultural differences
  assessment, 33
  documentation in medical
    records, 33
  findings, 33
  goals/outcomes, 33
  processes of care, 33

death, needs assessment. *See
    also* imminent death
  case managers
    after death, 14
    few months before death, 12
    6 months or longer before
      death, 11
  chaplain
    after death, 14
    few months before death,
      12
    6 months or longer before
      death, 11

delirium. *See*
    confusion/delirium
denial
    assessment, 34
    documentation in medical
        record, 35
    by families, 11
    findings, 34
    goals/outcomes, 35
    home abuse, 19, 20
    IDT care plan, 35
    processes of care, 34
    substance abuse, 31
depression
    assessments, 82
    causes, 79
    change in body image, 23,
        24, 25
    documentation in medical
        record, 82
    evaluation, 79–80
    findings, 79
    goals/outcomes, 81
    IDT care plan, 82
    processes of care, 80–81
diarrhea and anorectal
    problems
    assessments, 85
    causes, 82
    documentation in medical
        record, 85
    findings, 82–83
    goals/outcomes, 84–85
    IDT care plan, 85
    pharmacotherapy, 83–84
    processes of care, 83–84
documentation in medical rec-
    ords (clinical pro-
    cesses/symptom
    management)
    abuse in homes, 21
    agitation and anxiety, 60
    air hunger (dyspnea), 55–56
    anorexia and cachexia, 63
    belching and burping, 65
    bleeding, oozing,
        malodorous lesions, 70
    confusion/delirium, 73–74
    constipation, 76
    controlled substances,
        misuse/abuse, 32
    coughing, 78
    denial, 35
    depression, 82
    diarrhea/anorectal
        problems, 85
    dysphagia and
        oropharyngeal problems,
        87–88
    edema (ascites,
        lymphedema), 90
    fatigue, weakness, excessive
        sedation, 93

fatigue, weakness
    (aesthenia), excessive
    sedation, 93
fever and diaphoresis, 95
hiccups, 97
home safety, 44
imminent death, 100
nausea and vomiting, 108
pain, 127
pruritus, 130
seizures, 132
skin breakdown
    (prevention/treatment),
    140
spasms, skeletal
    muscle/bladder, 134–135
suicide,
    risk/prevention/coping
    with, 46
urinary problems, 142
xerostomia (dry mouth),
    144
do not (attempt to)
    resuscitate, 22
drug interactions, 154*t*
drug supplies, 42–43
drug therapy. *See*
    pharmacotherapy
dry mouth. *See* xerostomia
    (dry mouth)
durable power of attorney, 22
dysphagia and oropharyngeal
    problems
    assessment, 87
    causes, 85
    documentation in medical
        record, 87–88
    evaluation, 86
    findings, 85–86
    goals/outcomes, 87
    IDT care plan, 88
    processes of care, 86–87

edema (peripheral edema,
    ascites, lymphedema)
    assessments, 90
    causes, 88
    documentation in medical
        record, 90
    evaluation, 89
    findings, 88–89
    goals/outcomes, 90
    IDT care plan, 90
    processes of care, 89–90
effective/efficient care,
    principles, 3
environment/home safety,
    41–42
eructation. *See* belching and
    burping (eructation)
evaluation (clinical pro-
    cesses/symptom
    management)

agitation and anxiety, 57–58
anorexia and cachexia, 61
bleeding, oozing,
    malodorous lesions, 67
confusion/delirium, 71–72
constipation, 74–75
coughing, 77
depression, 79–80
diarrhea/anorectal
    problems, 83
dysphagia and
    oropharyngeal problems,
    86
edema (ascites,
    lymphedema), 89
fatigue, weakness, excessive
    sedation, 91–92
fever and diaphoresis, 94
hiccups, 95–96
imminent death, 98
insomnia/nocturnal
    restlessness, 101–102
nausea and vomiting,
    105–106
pain, 110–113
pruritus, 128
seizures, 131
skin breakdown
    (prevention/treatment),
    135–136
spasms, skeletal
    muscle/bladder, 133
urinary problems, 141
xerostomia (dry mouth),
    143

families
    changes in dynamics
        assessments, 26
        findings, 25–26
        goals/outcomes, 27
        processes of care, 26–27
        documentation, 15
    dynamics of
        assessment, 26
        documentation in medical
            record, 27
        documentation/medical
            record, 27
        findings, 25–26
        goals/outcomes, 27
        processes of care, 26–27
    needs assessment
        after death, 14
        few months before death,
            12
        last few days/weeks, 13
        6 months or longer before
            death, 11
fatigue, weakness (aesthenia),
    excessive sedation
    assessments, 93
    causes, 91

fatigue (*continued*)
documentation in medical
record, 93
evaluation, 91–92
findings, 91
goals/outcomes, 92–93
IDT care plan, 93
pharmacotherapy, 92
processes of care, 92
fever and diaphoresis
assessment, 95
causes, 93
documentation in medical
record, 95
evaluation, 94
findings, 93–94
goals/outcomes, 94
IDT care plan, 95
processes of care, 94
finances
assessment, 7f, 24, 40
findings, 40
processes of care, 28, 40–41
findings
advance care planning and
directives, 21
body image, changes in,
23–24
categorizations of, 4
completion of worldly
business/life closure, 28
denial, 34
family dynamics, changes in,
25–26
grief reactions, 35
living environment, finances,
support systems, 40
loss of independence, 23–24
findings (clinical pro-
cesses/symptom
management)
agitation and anxiety, 56–57
air hunger (dyspnea), 51
anorexia and cachexia, 61
bleeding, oozing,
malodorous lesions,
66–67
confusion/delirium, 71
constipation, 74
coughing, 77
depression, 79
diarrhea/anorectal
problems, 82–83
dysphagia and
oropharyngeal problems,
85–86
edema (ascites,
lymphedema), 88–89
fatigue, weakness, excessive
sedation, 91
fever and diaphoresis, 93–94
hiccups, 95
imminent death, 97–98

insomnia/nocturnal
restlessness, 101
nausea and vomiting, 105
pain, 110
pruritus, 128
seizures, 130–131
skin breakdown
(prevention/treatment),
135
spasms, skeletal
muscle/bladder, 133
urinary problems, 141
xerostomia (dry mouth),
143
fire safety, 41
functional hospice IDT, 7–8

goals and outcomes, 5
abuse in homes, 20–21
advance care
planning/healthcare
directives, 23
completion of worldly
business/life closure, 30
cultural differences, 33
denial, 35
family dynamics, 27
fatigue, weakness, excessive
sedation, 92–93
home safety, 44
suicide,
risk/prevention/coping
with, 46
goals and outcomes (clinical
processes/symptom
management)
agitation and anxiety, 60
air hunger (dyspnea), 55
anorexia and cachexia, 63
belching and burping
(eructation), 65
bleeding, oozing,
malodorous lesions,
69–70
confusion/delirium, 73
constipation, 76
coughing, 78
depression, 81
diarrhea/anorectal
problems, 84–85
dysphagia and
oropharyngeal problems,
87
edema (ascites,
lymphedema), 90
fever and diaphoresis, 94
hiccups, 97
imminent death, 100
insomnia/nocturnal
restlessness, 104
nausea and vomiting, 108
pain, 127
pruritus, 129

seizures, 132
skin breakdown
(prevention/treatment),
139
spasms, skeletal
muscle/bladder, 134
urinary problems, 142
xerostomia (dry mouth),
144
grief reactions
assessment, 36
in children, 38t–39t
documentation in medical
record, 37
findings, 35–36
goals/outcomes, 37
processes of care, 36–37
guardianship, 22

hiccups
assessments, 97
causes, 95
documentation in medical
record, 97
evaluation, 95–96
findings, 95
goals/outcomes, 97
IDT care plan, 97
pharmacotherapy, 96
processes of care, 96–97
home health aide. *See*
CNA/HHA
home safety
documentation in medical
records, 44
environment, 41–42
goals/outcomes, 44
medical supplies, 42–43
human experience, dimensions
of
biomedical, 6
practical, 6
psychosocial, 6
spiritual, 6

imminent death, 12, 13, 27, 56
assessments, 100
evaluation, 98
findings, 97–98
goals/outcomes, 100
IDT care plan, 100
pharmacotherapy, 99
processes of care, 98–100
independence, loss of. *See*
body image, changes/loss of
independence
infectious waste, 43
insomnia and nocturnal
restlessness
assessments, 104
causes, 101
documentation in medical
record, 104

evaluation, 101–102
findings, 101
goals/outcomes, 104
IDT care plan, 100
pharmacotherapy, 103–104
processes of care, 102–104
interdisciplinary teams (IDTs)
accountability for
documentation, 18
characteristics, 7–8
composition, 8
needs assessment
after death, 14–15
few months before death,
12–14
6 months (or longer)
before death, 11–12
notes/care plan, 5
optimal level, maintenance
of, 8
interdisciplinary teams (IDTs),
care plans
agitation/anxiety, 60
air hunger (dyspnea), 55
anorexia/cachexia, 63
belching/burping, 65
changes in family dynamics,
27
completion of worldly
business/life closure, 30
confusion/delirium, 74
constipation, 76
coughing, 78
denial, 35
depression, 82
diarrhea/anorectal
problems, 85
dysphagia/oropharyngeal
problems, 88
edema, ascites,
lymphedema, 90
fatigue, weakness, excessive
sedation, 93
fever/diaphoresis, 95
grief support, 37
hiccups, 97
home safety, 44
imminent death, 100
insomnia/nocturnal
restlessness, 100
malodorous lesions, 70
nausea/vomiting, 108
pain, 127
pruritus, 130
seizures, 132
skin breakdown, 140
spasms, bladder/skeletal
muscle, 135
substance abuse/misuse,
32
suicide/risk prevention, 47
urinary problems, 142
xerostomia, 144

ketamine protocol
background, 156
cautions, 157
continuous IV/SC infusion
protocol
adjuvant bedside
medications, 158–159
equipment, 158
contraindications, 156
guidelines for use (SV/IV or
oral), 157–158
indications, 156
monitoring, required,
158
pharmacy notes, 159
side effects, potential
general, 157
treatment exclusions,
relative, 157

lesions, malodorous. See
bleeding, oozing,
malodorous lesions
life closure. See worldly
business/life closure,
completion of
living environment,
assessment, 40
findings, 40
processes of care, 40–41
living will, 22
lymphedema. See edema
(peripheral edema, ascites,
lymphedema)

malodorous lesions. See
bleeding, oozing,
malodorous lesions
Medical Research Council
trials (Great Britain),
148
medication. See
pharmacotherapy

NA (Narcotics Anonymous),
31
NARANON (12 Step
Program), 31
nausea and vomiting
assessments, 108
causes, 105
documentation in medical
record, 108
evaluation, 105–106
findings, 105
goals/outcomes, 108
IDT care plan, 108
pharmacotherapy, 106–107
processes of care, 106–107
needle/syringe supplies, 43
needs over time
determination. See death,
needs assessment

nocturnal restlessness. See
insomnia and nocturnal
restlessness

oozing. See bleeding, oozing,
malodorous lesions
outdoor safety, 42

pain
assessments, 127
causes, 109
documentation in medical
record, 127
evaluation, 110–113
findings, 110
goals/outcomes, 127
IDT care plan, 127
pharmacotherapy, 114–125
processes of care, 113–126
palliative performance scale
(PPS), 162
palliative radiation therapy,
145–149
benefits/burdens, 147
ethical guiding principles,
146
fractionation
acute toxicity, 148
bone pain, 147
brain metastases, 148
dysuria/urinary frequency,
149
fatigue, 148
non-small cell lung-cancer,
148
skin symptoms, 148–149
visceral symptoms, 149
indications for, 146–147
patients, needs assessment
few months before death,
12
last few days/weeks, 13
6 months or longer before
death, 11
pharmacotherapy
agitation/anxiety, 58–59
air hunger (dyspnea), 53
anorexia/cachexia, 62
belching and burping
(eructation), 65
bladder spasms, 133
confusion/delirium, 72
constipation, 75–76
diarrhea/anorectal
problems, 83–84
drug interactions, 154t
dysphagia/oropharyngeal
problems, 86–87
fatigue, weakness, excessive
sedation, 92
general principles, 153–154
hiccups, 96
imminent death, 99

pharmacotherapy (*continued*)
    insomnia/nocturnal
        restlessness, 103–104
    nausea and vomiting,
        106–107
    pain, 114–125
    pruritus, 128–129
    seizures, 131–132
    skeletal muscle spasms, 134
physician, needs assessment
    after death, 14
    few months before death,
        12
    last few days/weeks, 13
    6 months or longer before
        death, 11
physicians order for life-
    sustaining treatment
    (POLST), 22
power of attorney, 22
processes of care, 5
    abuse in homes, 20
    advance care planning and
        directives, 22
    completion of worldly
        business/life closure,
        28–30
    cultural differences, 33
    denial, 34
    family dynamics, 26–27
    goals/outcomes, 37
    grief reactions, 35–36
    living environment, finances,
        support systems, 40–41
    suicide,
        risk/prevention/coping
        with, 45–46
processes of care (clinical pro-
    cesses/symptom
    management)
    agitation and anxiety, 58–60
    air hunger (dyspnea), 52–55
    anorexia and cachexia,
        62–63
    belching and burping
        (eructation), 65
    bladder spasms, 133–134
    bleeding, oozing,
        malodorous lesions,
        68–69
    confusion/delirium, 72–73
    constipation, 75–76
    coughing, 78
    depression, 80–81
    diarrhea/anorectal
        problems, 83–84
    dysphagia and
        oropharyngeal problems,
        86–87
    edema (ascites,
        lymphedema), 89–90
    fatigue, weakness, excessive
        sedation, 92

fever and diaphoresis, 94
hiccups, 96–97
imminent death, 98–100
insomnia/nocturnal
    restlessness, 102–104
nausea and vomiting,
    106–107
pain, 113–126
pruritus, 128–129
seizures, 131–132
skeletal muscle spasms, 134
skin breakdown
    (prevention/treatment),
    136–139
urinary problems, 141–142
xerostomia (dry mouth),
    143–144
pruritus
    assessments, 130
    causes, 128
    documentation in medical
        record, 130
    evaluation, 128
    findings, 128
    goals/outcomes, 129
    IDT care plan, 130
    pharmacotherapy, 128–129
    processes of care, 128–129

radiation therapy. *See*
    palliative radiation therapy
Radiation Therapy Oncology
    Group clinical trials, 148
rectal problems. *See* diarrhea
    and anorectal problems
resuscitation. *See* do not
    (attempt to) resuscitate
RN, needs assessment
    after death, 14
    few months before death,
        12
    last few days/weeks, 13
    6 months or longer before
        death, 11

safety issues. *See also* home
    safety
    confusion/delirium, 70, 72
    denial, 34, 35
    depression, 80
    education about, 20, 40,
        41–44
    home abuse assessment, 19
    insomnia/nocturnal
        restlessness, 102
    plan development, 20
sedation, excessive. *See*
    fatigue, weakness
    (aesthenia), excessive
    sedation
seizures
    assessments, 132
    causes, 130

documentation in medical
    record, 132
evaluation, 131
findings, 130–131
goals/outcomes, 132
IDT care plan, 132
pharmacotherapy, 131–132
processes of care, 131–132
sexual dysfunction, 24
skeletal muscle spasms. *See*
    spasms, skeletal
    muscle/bladder
skin breakdown
    (prevention/treatment)
    assessments, 140
    causes, 135
    documentation in medical
        record, 140
    evaluation, 135–136
    findings, 135
    goals/outcomes, 139,
        139*t*–140*t*
    IDT care plan, 140
    processes of care, 136–139
social worker, needs
    assessment
    after death, 15
    few months before death,
        13
    last few days/weeks, 14
    6 months or longer before
        death, 11–12
spasms, skeletal
    muscle/bladder
    causes, 133
    documentation in medical
        record, 134–135
    evaluation, 133
    findings, 133
    goals/outcomes, 134
    IDT care plan, 135
    pharmacotherapy, 133–134
    processes of care
        bladder spasms, 133–134
        skeletal muscle spasms, 134
stair/passageway safety, 42
substance abuse. *See*
    controlled substances,
    misuse/abuse
suicide. *See also* assisted death
    ideation/thoughts of, 19, 24,
        36, 44, 46
    IDT care plan, 47
    risk, prevention, coping with
        assessments, 45
        documentation in medical
            record, 47
        findings, 44–45
        goals/outcomes, 46
        processes of care, 45–46
support systems
    abuse in home, 19
    assessment, 40

body image/loss of independence, 24
findings, 40
grief reactions, 36
home safety, 44
processes of care, 40–41
symptom management. *See* clinical processes/symptom management

team meetings, 2*f*, 8, 9–10, 11
12 Step Programs, 31

urinary problems
assessments, 142
causes, 140–141
documentation in medical record, 142
evaluation, 141

findings, 141
goals/outcomes, 142
IDT care plan, 142
processes of care, 141–142

volunteers
choice of, with appropriate cultural values, 33
coordination of, 11, 12, 13, 15, 40, 73
needs assessment
after death, 15
few months before death, 13
6 months or longer before death, 12

weakness (aesthenia). *See* fatigue, weakness (aesthenia), excessive sedation

will, living, 22
worldly business/life closure, completion of
assessment, 28
documentation/medical records, 30
findings, 28
process of care, 28–30

xerostomia (dry mouth)
assessments, 144
causes, 143
documentation in medical record, 144
evaluation, 143
findings, 143
goals/outcomes, 144
IDT care plan, 144
processes of care, 143–144